Rashtriya Swasthya Bima Yojna

Rashtriya Swasthya Bima Yojna

Dr Harinder Singh
Dr Amandeep Kaur Shahi

KALPAZ

ISBN: 978-93-5128-223-5

Price: ₹ 790

First Published, 2017

Published by

Kalpaz Publications
C-30, Satyawati Nagar,
Delhi – 110052
E-mail: kalpaz@hotmail.com
Ph.: 9212142040

Printed at: G. Print Process, Delhi

Cataloging in Publication Data—DK
Courtesy: D.K. Agencies (P) Ltd. <docinfo@dkagencies.com>

Harinder Singh *(Professor of management studies)*, **author.**
Rasthriya Swasthya Bima Yojnaa / Dr Harinder Singh, Dr Amandeep Kaur Shahi.
pages cm
ISBN 9789351282235

1. Rashtriya Swasthya Bima Yojana (Program). 2. Health insurance—India. 3. Poor—Services for—India. I. Shahi, Amandeep Kaur, author. II. Title.

HG9399.I4S53 2016 DDC 368.4200954 23

Contents

Introduction

The book "Rashtriya Swasthya Bima Yojna" attempts to impart knowledge in the direction of provision of quality healthcare to the poor. The basic objective of the book is to examine the implementation of Rashtriya Swasthya Bima Yojna across country. More specifically, the objectives are (1) To work out the implementation and Impact of Rashtriya Swasthya Bima Yojna in various states of India; (2) To analyse comparative performance of Rashtriya Swasthya Bima Yojna with other public sector health insurance schemes; (3) To study the problems faced by Government Sponsored Health Insurance Schemes in India; and (4) To draw policy implications from the empirical analysis.The contents of the book are exhaustive and cover a variety of topics on the implementation and impact of Rashtriya Swasthya Bima Yojna in various states of India.

Foreword

Health Insurance is a kind of protection that provides benefits of payments for covered sickness or injury. It may be provided through a government-sponsored social health insurance programme or through private health insurance companies. Health Insurance can be purchased either on group basis by a firm to cover its employees or by individual consumers. In each case, the covered groups or individuals pay premium to protect themselves from high or unexpected healthcare expenses. Similar benefits for medical expenses can also be provided through social welfare programmes funded by the government. RSBY is an attempt to provide health insurance to low income BPL households and is being implemented by different states across India to protect them from major health shocks.

Many studies have been undertaken to examine implementation and impact of Rashtriya Swasthya Bima Yojna across country. The major studies on the subject include the works of Sunil Nagpal, Narayan Devadasan, Nishant Jain, David Dror, Sukumar Vellakal, Gerard La Forgia, Somil Nagpal, Robert Palacios, Vinod Vyasulu, Anil Swarup, Smriti Vashisht, Niraj Pandit, Kinnary Desai, Rajeev Ahuja and Rupalee Ruchismita who have highlighted the implementation and impacts of Rashtriya Swasthya Bima Yojna.

The present book by Dr Amandeep Kaur Shahi and Dr Harinder Singh is an endeavour in this direction and it deals with the contemporary issues and problems of Rashtriya Swasthya Bima Yojna. The book provides a thorough treatment of the subject, emphasising the important aspects of RSBY and covers its implementation and impact in various states of India. The work is based on secondary data and has been structured into five chapters. Each chapter in the book contains a set of objectives and analysis.

Statistical techniques like tabular analysis, ratios, percentages, averages, co-efficients of variation, pie-charts, bar-diagrammes etc.

have been applied to analyse the data for achieving the desired objectives. The study highlights the impact of RSBY on the below poverty line (BPL) population in 30 states of India.To study the impact of RSBY on BPL population of India, the study focused on four key performance indicators (KPIs) viz. Claims Ratio (utilisation by beneficiaries), Conversion Ratio (a tool for measuring outreach), Hospitalisation Ratio (an indicator of utilisation of healthcare) and Total Expense Ratio (a parameter to judge the profit to the insurance companies). These KPIs have been analysed from aggregated state level and insurer-wise data for the first year of operations for 24 states and 10 insurers, for the second year for 17 states and 10 insurers and for the third year for 5 states and 4 insurers. The comparison of government sponsored health insurance schemes (GSHISs) has also been studied.

There have been around 7.16 million hospitalisation cases from BPL families from the year 2008. In January 2014, total 30 states/ UTs have enrolled with RSBY and the total BPL families were 77.80 million, out of which 40.13 million families (51.6 per cent) have enrolled with the RSBY. The results revealed that the first year under the RSBY was a period for experience gain and the scheme and processes there under were gradually stabilising but there was still much to be done. An appraisal of the scheme attempted on the basis of experience gained in second and third round focused to acknowledge that the scheme has indeed been successful. It comes into light that RSBY is giving a positive impact, as more and more BPL population is getting registered and availing the benefits from the scheme over time. The RSBY scheme is a supportive mechanism to BPL population and number of other developing countries follow this effective scheme.

The government sponsored health insurance schemes (GSHISs) have been compared on the basis of implementation, coverage, sources of finance, premium, benefit packages and empanellment of network hospitals. In regard to comparison of government sponsored health insurance schemes, the number of people benefitting from health insurance has gone up appreciably over the years under the aegis of Rashtriya Swasthya Bima Yojna, Rajiv Aarogyasri, Vajpayee Arogyasri and Kalaignar health insurance scheme implemented by the union and state governments.The comparison of government sponsored health insurance schemes showed that RSBY provided the wide range of hospitalisation benefits to the beneficiaries across India.

On the whole this study provides a comprehensive understanding of health insurance in India. The recommendations are insightful and need to be carefully examined by the policymakers at the central and state levels when designing future strategies. It provides detailed comparative analysis of government sponsored health insurance schemes and is a source of information and inspiration for those who work in the area of health insurance.

I congratulate to Dr Amandeep Kaur Shahi and Dr Harinder Singh for bringing out such an up-to-date and immensely useful book for the students, teachers, researchers, policymakers and those interested in the field of health insurance in general and RSBY, in particular.

Dr R.S. Bawa
Vice-chancellor
Chandigarh University
Gharuan, Punjab, India

Acknowledgements

It gives us great pleasure in expressing our gratitude to all those people who have supported us and had their contributions in writing this book. First and foremost, we must acknowledge and thank the Almighty God for blessing, protecting and guiding us throughout this period. We could never have accomplished this without the faith we have in the Almighty.

We also take this opportunity to thank Dr Narayan Devadasan, Director, Institute of Public Health, Bangalore, who laid seeds of enthusiasm and passion in our pursuit of knowledge.

We are thankful to Dr Nishant Jain, Deputy Programme Director, Indo-German Social Society Programme, Deutsche Gesellschaftfur Internationale Zusammenarbeit (GIZ) GmbH and Ministry of Health and Family Welfare, New Delhi, Ms. Heena Dhawan, Deutsche Gesellschaftfür Internationale Zusammenarbeit (GIZ) GmbH for their constant support, guidance and immensely valuable insights throughout the book writing. We are and shall remain indebted to Dr Nishant Jain from the bottom of our heart for his whole hearted guidance, constant support and encouragement in completing this work. We sincerely feel that it would have been possible for us to bring this work into the current shape without his commendable and inspired guidance.

We shall be failing in our duty if we do not express our gratitude to all our family members who constantly encouraged us. We would have never reached this stage without their help and kind cooperation. We shall remain indebted towards them forever for their immense love and support.

Lastly, we also take this opportunity to thank all our friends and colleagues who have helped and encouraged us in writing this book.

We thank them all and the others who genuinely offered us help. We appreciate everyone whom we have thanklessly missed to remember and have contributed towards completion of the work.

Dr Harinder Singh

Dr Amandeep Kaur Shahi

List of Abbreviations

ACCORD - Action for Community Organisation Rehabilitation and Development
AP - Andhra Pradesh
BPL - Below Poverty Line
CBIEC - Capacity Building and Information Education Communication
CGHI - Central Government Health Insurance
CHI - Community Health Insurance
CII - Confederation of Indian Industry
CMKHIS - Chief Minister Kalaignar Health Insurance Scheme
ESIS - Employee State Insurance Scheme
GDP - Gross Domestic Premium
GSHI - Government Sponsored Health Insurance
GSHISs - Government Sponsored Health Insurance Schemes
GOI - Government of India
HCFP - Health Care for the Poor Programme
HP - Himachal Pradesh
IAS - Indian Administrative Service
IDPM - Institutional Development and Project Management
IEC - Information and Education Campaign
ILO - Indian Labour Organisation
IPH - Institute of Public Health
IRDA - Insurance Regulatory Development Authority
IT - Information Technology
ITT - Intention to Treat
J&K - Jammu and Kashmir

KPIs - Key Performance Indicators
LIC - Life Insurance Corporation
MIS - Management Information System
M&E - Monitoring and Evaluation
MFIs - Micro Finance Institutions
MP - Madhya Pradesh
MOHFW - Ministry of Health and Family Welfare
MOLE - Ministry of Labour and Employment
NACO - National AIDS Control Organisation
NABH - National Accreditation Board for Hospitals
NCCC - Nandana Critical Care Centre
NHS - National Health Service
NHP - National Health Package
NHIS - National Health Insurance Scheme
NRHM - National Rural Health Mission
NURHM - National Urban Rural Health Mission
NSS - National Sample Survey
NREGA - National Rural Employment Guarantee Scheme
NSSO - National Sample Survey Office
OECD - Organisation for Economic Co-operation and Development
OOP - Out-of-Pocket
OPD - Out-patient Department
PHI - Private Health Insurance
PHFI - Public Health Foundation of India
PPP - Public Private Partnership
PPP - Purchasing Power Parity
PTE - Pure Technical Efficiency
RAS - Rajiv Aarogyasri Scheme
RSBY - Rashtriya Swasthya Bima Yojna
SEWA - Self- Employed Women's Association
SHI - Social Health Insurance
SHH - Students Health Home

SNA	- State Nodal Agency
TNHSS	- Tamil Nadu Health System Society
TPAs	- Third Party Administrators
TOT	- Treatment on Treated
UHC	- Universal Health Coverage
UHIS	- Universal Health Insurance Scheme
UTs	- Union Territories
VAS	- Vajpayee Arogyasri Scheme
WHO	- World Health Organisation

Chapter - 1

Introduction

Insurance is "a technique for financing risks by combining a sufficient number of loss exposure units to make the loss predictable" (Outreville, 1998). The history of insurance can be traced with the establishment of a British company called the Oriental Life Insurance Company, which started in Calcutta in 1818, Bombay Assurance Company (1823) and the Madras Equitable Life Insurance Society in (1829) (Sinha, 2004). These companies operated in India but were not able to insure the Indian people and give the insurance protection only to the health of Europeans residing in different states of India. The British started and administered the first general insurance company in 1850 known as Triton Insurance Company Ltd. Indian Mercantile Insurance Company Limited established in Bombay in 1907 was the first indigenous general insurance company (Sinha, 2005). The wholly Indian-owned insurance company, namely, New India Assurance Company Limited was incorporated on July 23, 1919 which commenced its operations in October the same year (Narayanan, 2006). There was no exclusive legislation to govern the activities of insurance companies during the nineteenth century. To control the operations of life insurance in India, the Indian Life Insurance Companies Act, 1912 was enacted. However, the first insurance regulations were came into existence with the passing of Indian Insurance Act, 1938. The Act made provision for required equity capital to carry out insurance business, ceiling on shareholding pattern, strict control on investments, agency commission etc. Subsequently, a separate wing was established in the Ministry of Finance to administer the provisions under the Act (Sharma and Agarwal, 2005).

In the context of the development of insurance and health insurance in India, it has been categorised under two stages. Stage I depicts the development before liberalisation of insurance sector and stage II represents the development after the liberalisation period of insurance in India.

Table 1.1: Development of Insurance and Health Insurance in India (Chronology: 1912- 2013)

Year	***Development***
	STAGE-I
1912	Insurance Act, 1912 passed, setting down rules and regulations specific to Indian insurance industry (IRDA, 2007).
1923	Workman's Compensation Act passed, which provide workmen and their dependents some relief in case of accidents arising out of or in the course of employment, causing death or disablement (NIFHW).
1938	Insurance Act, 1938 passed, recognised two insurance categories, i.e. life and non-life (general) insurance (IRDA, 2007).
1948	Employee's State Insurance (ESI) Act passed, providing protection to workers and dependents in the organised sector for sickness, maternity and death (Mavalankar and Bhat, 2000).
1954	The Central Government Health Scheme started in 1954, providing health cover to employees of Central Government (retired also), MPs, Judges, Freedom Fighters and their families (Public Health Foundation of India, 2011).
1956	Life insurance industry nationalised and Life Insurance Corporation of India (LIC) set up subsequently (IRDA, 2007).
1968	The Tariff Advisory Committee was established up this year (Sinha, 2005).
1972	General Insurance industry was nationalised (www.irda.gov.in).
1986	General Insurance Corporation of India (GIC) introduced Mediclaim insurance policy (Devadasan and Nandraj, 2006).
1994	Malhotra committee submitted its report and recommended the entry of the private sector in the insurance segment and the foreign companies can be allowed by floating Indian companies, preferably as joint ventures with Indian partners (Sinha, 2012).
1999	Insurance Regulatory and Development Authority (IRDA) Act was passed (Shijith and Shekar, 2011).
	STAGE-II
2000	General Insurance Corporation (GIC) became the national re-insurer (IRDA, 2007).
2001	Third Party Administrators (TPAs) system introduced health insurance (Bhat and Babu, 2003).

2002	The Insurance Regulatory and Development Authority (Protection of Policyholder's Interests) Regulations, 2002 was passed to safeguard the Interest of the policyholder (IRDA Protection of Policyholders' Interest, 2002).
2003	Establishment of National health insurance working group (IRDA, 2003-04).
2003	Universal Health Insurance Scheme (UHIS) introduced (GOI, 2011).
2006	First standalone health insurance company commenced business this year (IRDA, 2012).
2007	The Indian Insurance market was de-tariffed (Krishnan, 2007).
2008	Rashtriya Swasthya Bima Yojna (RSBY) started rolling in India from 1st April 2008 (www.rsby.gov.in)
2008	Insurance Information Bureau set up by IRDA (primarily working on health and motor data) (IRDA, 2009-10).
2009	The renewability of health insurance policies (IRDA, 2007).
2010	The Preferred Provider Network (PPN) of hospitals was introduced in July 2010 to offer cashless medical treatment (IRDA, 2007).
2011	Portability of health insurance policies have been started by IRDA (Annual reports, IRDA, 2011-12).
2012	The Health Insurance Forum has been constituted (Annual reports, 2011-12).
2013	IRDA issued guidelines on standardisation in health insurance (Guidelines on Standardisation, 2013).
2013	Insurance Repository System has been established (Handbook on Insurance repository, 2013).

1.1 Health Insurance

The term health has been derived from the term hale which means "wholeness, a being whole, sound or well". Way back in 1948, World Health Organisation defined the term as "a state of complete physical, mental and social well-being and not merely the absence of disease or infirmity". The health insurance connotes a kind of insurance that makes payment for the patient's medical expenditure. Sometimes it includes coverage of disability, nursing for longer periods etc. Such a provision is either under some government ranged programme or guaranteed by a private insurance company (Rajan and Dhunna, 2002). For any person health is of paramount importance for a person and his family. This deserves to be taken care of priority basis. Since healthy citizens make a healthy nation over a longer period of time. Insurance means reduction of financial and health risk to every member of a group who opt for health insurance. The fund so raised from the premium of all members is utilised to compensate an unfortunate follow in the group. Insurance is such a boon which boosts an insurer's morale that an ailment cannot destabilise him economically and health-wise. With the result the policyholder can faced the challenges posed by life hopefully. The basic principle underlying insurance is that anyone can suffer health in society. The danger of loss of health looms large on every day.

Health insurance is a system in which insurers in a way that by making a small prepayment and pooling of resources. Many people can meet their challenges of ill health with fortitude and courage. A healthy man does not mind for paying a small amount for the sake of his health. Small contributions received from a very wide based result into very large pool of funds that can be utilised to provide health cover to the insured.

Countries across the world are introducing demand-side health financing mechanisms. The main feature of these initiatives is that money follows the demand and that it is not linked to the supply side of healthcare. In simple terms, hospitals earn money based on the demand, which is raised by the population and not by getting a fixed amount from the government. For example, in Thailand, once a person is enrolled in one of the three main schemes of the country, then he/she can visit any network health facility to get free treatment. Similar mechanisms exist in many other developing countries such as Philippines, Indonesia, Ghana, etc. The income of the health facility depends on the number of persons choosing that facility for treatment. Recognising the limitations of focusing only on the supply-side model, in the last few years, the Government of India has introduced various demand-side financing mechanisms to provide financial security for the vulnerable segments of the society. One of the first initiatives in this direction was a health insurance called Universal Health Insurance Scheme (UHIS) launched by the Ministry of Finance in 2003. This scheme provided coverage to beneficiaries with a limit and was implemented by the public sector insurance companies. Another set of schemes was launched by the different state governments. These initiatives were novel and the intention was to provide health insurance to the vulnerable sections of the population of the state. However, most of these initial set of schemes were not able to achieve the desired objectives and were closed after operations of one or two years.

State-level health insurance schemes launched by the states of Punjab, Kerala, Assam, etc. during 2005–07 are some of the examples. Though the intention to provide health insurance by these schemes was laudable and much needed, these schemes were not successful in reaching the desired objectives due to many reasons. The basic model of these schemes was to hire an insurance company and provide that insurance company with money based on the estimated number of families to be covered. Subsequently, it was the responsibility of the selected insurance companies to carry out each step of the implementation. Since all of these schemes had no enrollment process, i.e. the beneficiary families were automatically enrolled in the scheme if they had below poverty line (BPL) card/ration card, etc. Awareness generation was a critical element and most often people were not even aware that they are now covered by an insurance scheme. In addition to this, there was no institution within the government that was responsible for full-time management of these schemes. The premium was paid in lump-sum, based on the targeted population to the insurance companies. Even the benefit package was not always most useful. For example, in the benefit package of one of the states, high-end diseases like Alzheimer's and Parkinson's were included, but simple diseases that are more frequent were not covered. In this scenario, there was no incentive for the insurance companies to inform the beneficiaries about the schemes and inform them about using it. Therefore, most of these schemes were closed by the respective state governments after one or two years of being in operation.

Rashtriya Swasthya Bima Yojna (RSBY) is initiated by the Ministry of Labour, Government of India in October 2007 and it became operational from 1st April 2008, aimed to cover the unorganised sector in India. It is an attempt to provide health insurance to low income BPL households and is being implemented by different states across India and protects them from major health shocks. In 2007, the Government of Andhra Pradesh launched a health insurance scheme called Rajiv Aarogyasri that focused on providing coverage to mostly tertiary care. The argument of the state government in introducing a tertiary care health insurance scheme was that the government facilities provided for good quality, free of cost secondary care. But access to quality tertiary care was lacking in the state and therefore, it was being provided through this health insurance scheme. Even though the decision to provide only tertiary care is controversial and a revised definition of BPL for this scheme covered more than 80 per cent of the population of the state, this scheme for the first time went about designing and implementation in a very methodical manner. A separate institution called Aarogyasri Trust was set up for the implementation of the scheme. This scheme used Information Technology (IT) very effectively whereby electronic claims were transferred from hospitals to the insurance company on a regular basis. A very close co-operation was developed between the Aarogyasri Trust and the implementing insurance company. This resulted in successful implementation of the scheme. Critics argue that though this scheme has achieved success, the priorities of the state government are misplaced, where a disproportionately large percentage of the health budget is being spent on a scheme providing only tertiary care. The scheme has revised its benefit package so as to even include some of the secondary care diseases, but it continues to face challenges like moral hazards, appropriate targeting and increasing costs. Aarogyasri inspired a few other state governments, e.g. Karnataka, Tamil Nadu, Maharashtra and Gujarat, to initiate similar tertiary care schemes. The main feature of most of these health insurance schemes was Public-Private Partnership (PPP) model where schemes were funded by the government in the sense that the premium on behalf of the beneficiaries was paid by the government to the insurance companies which were responsible for the implementation of the scheme. In some of the states, e.g. Karnataka's Vajpayee Aarogyasri Scheme, the state government decided to park the funds with a government-owned trust instead of an insurance company. The Trust implemented the scheme directly, which included informing the beneficiaries and entering into arrangements with hospitals for claim payments. In terms of provision of healthcare, also a mixed approach was adopted whereby a beneficiary could access both public and private healthcare facilities for treatment.

1.2 Pattern of Health Insurance

The health insurance expenditure can be dealt with along two channels. For instance, one can pay from pocket or alternatively state or society comes to ones help. Self financing is beyond the reach of many people in a poor country with little savings. As such a private health insurance policy as a better option than looking at friends, relatives or banks for assistance. In case of public financing either there are great sponsored medical care programme or social security arrangements or outright grants. In the current health insurance system, health insurance can broadly define into four main categories (1) Social Health Insurance; (2) Private Health Insurance; (3) Community Health Insurance; and (4) Government Sponsored Health Insurance.

(1) Social Health Insurance

Social health insurance (SHI) schemes are financed mainly through salaries of the employees which are based on the income or earnings. Social health insurance schemes are compulsory for the employees, workers of the particular categories. SHI Scheme is a fund organised by government with better benefits in return for contribution. It is mandatory for employees in the public and the premiums are fixed according to income but not as per the health risk. In this case the benefits are equal and payments contributions are according to spending on health services. The social health insurance includes the Central Government Health Scheme (CGHS) and Employees State Insurance Scheme (ESIS). CGHS was introduced in 1954 as a contributory scheme which provides health insurance to central government employees and their families. According to ESI Act 1948, Employee State Insurance Scheme covers employees against loss of wages due to improper work following sickness, maternity, disability and death due to employment injury. (Devadasan and Nandraj, 2006).

(2) Private Health Insurance

Private health insurance is a system which is optional from an insured and lucrative for the insurance companies. An insurance company is guided by profit motive and it receives premium from policyholders and make such investments to increase the insurance funds. In India, health insurance is synonymous with Mediclaim which was introduced in 1986 offered by government. In India, the existence of health insurance was in the year 1999. According to Insurance Regulatory Development Authority Bill, the insurance sector given the option to private and foreign participation and also give the permission in guidelines for the entry of private general insurance companies for dealing in health insurance business.With the coming of IRDA, there came regulations to ensure interest of insurance purchasers. In 2001, the provision was made for TPA's which were meant to provide a faster expansion and penetration of insurance sector as an industry.

(3) Community Health Insurance

Community Health Insurance (CHI) was started in 1952 in Kolkata. Community health insurance scheme is "any not-for-profit insurance scheme that is aimed primarily at the informal sector and formed on the basis of a collective pooling of health risks and in which the members participate in its management". Community Health Insurance programmes resolve around the payment of premium and collection of funds to meet the losses of health hazards. Learning large on the insured while framing products of these cost is taken in view that the interests of low income population are served and also the economic and social completion of segment, societies is taken care of because in a district or a town there live diverse classes of society. Generally such schemes moved by a hospital and aims at the service of the surrounding area. Presently there are about 20 CHI scheme in India, like Action for Community Organisation Rehabilitation and Development (ACCORD), Community health insurance scheme in Tamil Nadu, Karuna trust and Yeshvani scheme in Karnataka, Self Employed Women Association in Gujarat etc (Devadasan *et al.,* 2004).

(4) Government Sponsored Health Insurance

The government introduces a health insurance programme under Government Health Insurance Schemes (GHI) usually for the below poverty population. For the BPL population, in this programme the 100 per cent financed by the government from its revenues. The important GHI schemes are (a) Rashtriya Swasthya Bima Yojna, (b) Rajiv Aarogyasri Scheme (Andhra Pradesh), (c) Chief Minister Kalaignar's Health Insurance Scheme (Tamil Nadu), (d) Vajpayee Arogyasri Scheme (PHFI, 2011).

(a) Rashtriya Swasthya Bima Yojna

Rashtriya Swasthya Bima Yojna (RSBY) is initiated by the Ministry of Labour, Government of India in October 2007 and it became operational from 1st April 2008, aimed to cover the unorganised sector in India. It is an attempt to provide health insurance to low income

BPL households and is being implemented by different states across India and protects them from major health shocks. By paying a small amount of ₹ 30 for a five members family, the beneficiary will get a smart card wherein the details of the family are recorded in it. It is a valuable tool of the scheme as it is ensures cashless treatment of beneficiaries at the enlisted hospitals. The hospitals are paid for their services by the insurance companies. Subsequently insurance companies are selected through open bidding process with the condition that they will agree to the premium decide by the government on yearly basis. The subsidy is divided between central and state governments in the ratio of 3:1. State Government is advised to incorporate various benefits to Rashtriya Swasthya Bima Yojana (RSBY) beneficiaries. The state government has provided hospitalisation benefits at empanelled public and private hospitals up to a maximum of ₹ 30,000 per family per year. Hospitalisation expenses are meant for treatment of general ailments with as little exclusions as possible. If a person is already suffering from a disease it has to be covered under RSBY. Moreover the beneficiaries are entitled to travelling allowance with upper limit of ₹ 1000 and cap of ₹ 100 per visit. The scheme is managed by the insurer while it is monitored by a nodal agency setting by the state government having members from different state departments (Rashtriya Swasthya Bima Yojna, 2008). The Process flow for Rashtriya Swasthya Bima Yojana scheme is as:

- The state nodal agency is the body which is selected by state government for the administration and control of the districts;
- The requirements and tenders have to be given by the nodal agencies to insurance companies;
- Interested insurance companies fill the quotations and submit;
- To check and evaluate the bids and to choose the insurance company and further hospitals, smart card service providers and intermediaries;
- To make ready and submit the invitations to central government;
- Central government examines and select the proposal;
- A memorandum of understanding is done in the central and state government /nodal agency;

- Completion of memorandum of understanding in insurance companies and nodal agency;
- To assign the responsibilities of BPL population data to the insurance companies by government of concerned states; and
- To design the policies for delivery of smart cards by nodal agency/ state government in consultation with the insurance company (Swarup, 2008).

There was a five year plan for rolling out the RSBY which allows each participating state to contract 20 per cent of their respective districts each year. In 1st April 2008, the states like Delhi, Rajasthan, Gujarat, Haryana, Bihar, Uttrakhand, Kerala, Punjab, Chhattisgarh, Karnataka, Maharashtra, Tamil Nadu, Uttar Pradesh, West Bengal and Jharkhand have expressed its intention of joining the scheme. There are 30 states/ UTs enrolled with Rashtriya Swasthya Bima Yojna and approximately 40.13 million families enrolled with Rashtriya Swasthya Bima Yojna upto January 2014.[1] The target group in Rashtriya Swasthya Bima Yojna has found to be absolutely imperative in evolving a scheme that could have a meaningful impact. They are primarily-poor, self-employed illiterate, migratory and unskilled people. Thus, the scheme, had to be cashless, because there was no way in which the beneficiary could raise the financial resources and then claim reimbursement from any agency. The reimbursement process itself is normally so cumbersome that it would have been virtually impossible for those below poverty line, even if they could raise the resources upfront to claim the benefit. A large number of workers in India migrate from one state to the other in search of employment. So far, none of the health insurance schemes addresses this aspect. An added complexity emerges when only some in the family migrate and rest of them stay back. On account of illiteracy, repeated documentation cannot be resorted to and, in this sense, the cashless system was the only alternative (Swarup, 2008).

Enrollment of Beneficiaries

The enrollment of the beneficiaries will be undertaken by the Insurance Company selected by the State Government and approved by the Central Government. The Insurer shall enroll the BPL beneficiaries based on the soft data provided by the State Government/ Nodal Agency and issue smart card as per Central Government specifications through Smart Card Vender and handover the same to the beneficiaries at enrollment station/village level itself during the enrollment period. Further the enrollment process shall continue at designated centres agreed by the Government /Nodal Agency after the enrollment period is over to provide the smart card for remaining beneficiaries. Insurer in consultation with the State Government/ Nodal Agency shall chalk out the enrollment cycle upto village level in a manner that representative of Insurer, Government/Nodal Agency and smart card vender can complete the task in scheduled time. The process of enrollment shall be as under:

(a) The data relating to BPL families in the selected districts shall be entered into prescribed software by the concerned State Government/Nodal Agency.

(b) A soft and hard copy of this data shall be provided by the State Government/Nodal Agency to the Insurer selected by the State Government/Nodal Agency.

(c) The Insurer will arrange for preparation of the smart card as per the prescribed stipulation.

(d) A schedule of programme shall be worked out by the Government/Nodal Agency in consultation with the Insurer for each enrollment station/village in the district.

(e) Advance publicity of the visit of representatives of the State Government and the Insurance Provider shall be done by the State Government/Nodal Agency in respective villages.

(f) List of BPL should be posted prominently in the enrollment station/village by the Insurer.

(g) The representatives shall visit each enrollment station/village in the selected district jointly on the pre-schedule dates for the purpose of taking photograph of the head of the family and the thumb impression of the head of the family and the other eligible member of the family, enrollment and issuance of smart card.

(h) The softwares to be used by the Insurance Company for the purpose of enrollment and thereafter for the purpose of transaction at the hospitals and data transmission therefrom shall be the ones approved by the Central Government.

(i) At the time of enrollment, the government official shall identify each beneficiary in the presence of the insurance representative.

(j) At the time of handing over the card, the Insurer shall collect the registration fee of ₹ 30 from the beneficiary.

(k) This amount will be adjusted against the amount of premium to be paid to the Insurer by the Nodal Agency.

(l) The Insurer's representative shall also provide a pamphlet along with Smart Card to the beneficiary indicating the list of the networked hospitals, the availability of benefits and the names and details of the contact person/persons. To prevent damage to the smart card, a plastic jacket should be provided to keep the smart card.

(m) The beneficiary shall also be informed about the date on which the card will become operational (month).

(b) Rajiv Aarogyasri Scheme

Rajiv Aarogyasri Scheme (RAS) is a state funded health insurance scheme started in Andhra Pradesh during the year 2007 to provide risk cover for the poor households against costly medical and surgical procedures. Aarogyasri healthcare trust which is an autonomous body looks after the management of the scheme. Premium at the rate of ₹ 68 per person is paid to an insurance company by the state government where upon the company becomes responsible for provision of health insurance cover to beneficiaries (Institute of Public Health, 2009). It was in 2007 that this project was initiated in three districts on trial basis. Later, it was introduced in a phased manner in all the districts. Under the scheme each BPL household was given a white card as method to reach them (Yellaiah, 2013). The scheme envisages provision of ₹ 1.50 lakh per household per annum to meet the expenses of hospitalisation and surgery. This amount of ₹ 1.50 lakh can be used by a family collectively or individually to supplement this amount, another sum of ₹ 50,000 is paid to them to meet sundry expenses. The insurance policy is of one year duration. Hospitals are supposed to render primary healthcare to the insurer.

(c) Chief Minister Kalaignar Health Insurance Scheme

On the basis of success of RSBY (a central scheme), the

Government of Tamil Nadu launched Chief Minister Kalaignar health insurance scheme for life saving treatment in July 2009 which covers the medical risk with cashless transactions. People who have an annual income of less than ₹ 72,000 are eligible for the scheme and it provides sum insured of ₹ 1,00,000 per family for four years with yearly premium of 469 per family to be totally paid by the state government. In the listed hospitals patients can avail the medical facilities. The state government oversees and provides financial support to the scheme through its department of health. The state has entrusted Tamil Nadu Health Systems Society (TNHSS) to implementing the health insurance scheme.The Chief Minister Kalaignar health insurance scheme implemented jointly by Star Health and Allied Insurance Company.

(d) Vajpayee Arogyasri Scheme

Vajpayee Arogyasri Scheme (VAS) launched in 2010, provides similar tertiary coverage for the treatment of serious and life threatening ailments for the vulnerable segments of society (primarily people living below the poverty line). The state launched the VAS as a pilot in the seven districts in the Gulbarga division in the northern part of Karnataka state with the objective of covering all the eligible BPL population against health shocks caused by serious and high-cost ailments. The emphasis on tertiary care is a conscious attempt to compensate for its limited availability in public institutions and to enlist the substantial capacity available in the private sector. The VAS scheme offers cashless treatment for 402 listed procedures (and an additional 50 follow-up packages), providing a cover of ₹ 1.5 lakh to ₹ 2 lakh per insured family of five members free of cost with a dominant focus on those requiring major surgical interventions. The scheme was initiated primarily to protect the BPL population (Forgia and Nagpal, 2012).

The basic objective of the book is to examine the implementation of Rashtriya Swasthya Bima Yojna in India. The specific objectives were:

1. To work out the implementation and Impact of Rashtriya Swasthya Bima Yojna in various states of India;
2. To analyse comparative performance of Rashtriya Swasthya Bima Yojna with other public sector health insurance schemes;

3. To study the problems faced by Government Sponsored Health Insurance Schemes in India; and
4. To draw policy implications from the empirical analysis.

The book has been divided into seven chapters including the present one. Chapter II reviews the literature related to the study. Data sources and methodology for analysis are described in Chapter III. Chapter IV examines the implementation and impact of Rashtriya Swasthya Bima Yojna in various states of India. Chapter V analyses the comparative performance of Rashtriya Swasthya Bima Yojna with other public sector health insurance schemes. The problems of government sponsored health insurance schemes discuss in Chapter VI. Chapter VII contains summary, conclusion, along with policy implications derived from the study.

Note

1. www.rsby.gov.in

Chapter - 2

Rashtriya Swasthya Bima Yojna: An Inter State Analysis

It is generally believed that social security provision should be made for millions of families who are without regular resources to livelihood and thus lack social security. On Gandhi Jayanti, 2007, honourable Prime Minister Manmohan Singh announced Rashtriya Swasthya Bima Yojna (RSBY) for the welfare of rural landless labourers which was to be in the form of cash transfer for the poor of old age living below poverty line. The scheme in itself is the largest of its kinds in the world as hospitalisation coverage is ensured to about 7.16 million poor people in the under developed areas. It is not only the scale but also the approach for identification of beneficiaries is very reliable and far reaching (Jain, 2013). The objective of this chapter is to examine the implementation of Rashtriya Swasthya Bima Yojna and to determine the impact of Rashtriya Swasthya Bima Yojna on BPL people in various states of India. The chapter has been divided into five sections. Section I deals with health financing in India. Section II covers the implementation of RSBY in various states of India. The state-wise impact of RSBY on Below Poverty Line people has been undertaken in Section III. Section IV examines insurer-wise impact of RSBY on Below Poverty Line population. The whole discussion has been concluded in Section V.

In order to identify the impact, the chapter focused on four key performance indicators (KPIs) - Claims Ratio (utility to the beneficiaries), Conversion Ratio (to measure depth of outreach subject to the quality of the BPL list), Hospitalisation Ratio (to gauge utilisation) and Total Expense Ratio (to evaluate profitability to the insurer). These KPIs have been analysed from aggregated state level and insurer-wise data for the first year of operations for 24 states and 10 insurers, for the second year for 17 states and 10 insurers and for the third year for 5 states and 4 insurers.

SECTION - I

2.1 Health Financing in India

After independence Indian parliament enacted national health policy which aimed at providing health covers to masses. Health insurance scheme was amended later on in 2002. Funding of this scheme was borne by Government of India and different state governments. Since the population of country is very huge the funds made by the government has always remained insufficient for the purpose. As a result majority of Indians have to bear the cost of medical treatment for their own pockets. It is evident from National Health Accounts data that only 20 per cent of health expenditure is borne by government while almost the entire amount is paid by the individuals from their own pockets. Nowhere in the world is visible such a situation. A perusal of World Bank studies reveals that about 25 per cent of Indian population slips below the poverty line because of huge medical bills. Market for healthcare is without regulations and private health providers contributed about 77 per cent of healthcare system (Peters *et al.*, 2002). Government of India health spending has to be estimated to about 4.5 per cent of GDP while expenditure on healthcare is meagre 0.9 per cent of GDP (IRDA, 2013). Lack of funds, faulty infrastructure, low quality healthcare and poor accessibility to the rural people characterise public healthcare system.

Figures relating to rural population suggest that the highest monetary burden on the poor people's due to costly medicines and due to indoor treatment. As per estimates medicines accounted for 40 per cent of medical expenditure. Another estimate puts this figure at 75 per cent. This constituted 77 per cent for rural people and about 70 per cent for urban regions. However, for another estimate for claims that expenditure on medicines from patients pocket was 77 per cent in villages (Selvaraj and Nabar, 2010) and 69 per cent in urban areas (Garg and Karan, 2009). According to report indoor treatment of a low income person in villages cost ₹ 2,530 in a government hospital and ₹ 5,431 in a private hospital. It ranges between 10-25 times of one's monthly income. In this way hospitalisation leads to further impoverishment of poor people and brought them to the verge of bankruptcy (Peters *et al.*, 2002).

World Health Organisation estimates suggested that in 2007, private health expenditure was about 73.5 per cent of total healthcare expenditure in India. An overwhelming amount of 90 per cent came from the pocket of concerned individuals. Government contribution to healthcare system was just 26.5 per cent (WHO, 2010). About 94 per cent of Indian labour force is engaged with private unorganised sector. It presents a depressing spectacle that about 433 million labourers have to fend for themselves during an ailment. These people feel highly insecure because being poor they fall easy prey to illness and have to resort to medical care and treatment. It is a fact that health insurance can come to their help and save them from such heavy expenditures that further impoverishes them. Poor people have neither capability nor willingness and knowledge to go for health insurance cover. Keeping in view the size of Indian population, the health scenario become quite frightening. The government policy-makers caught in a par dodge because people are entitled to free treatment in government hospitals but the fact remains that free government health services are not sufficient enough for everybody. The gap between demand and supply results into expenditure from patients' pocket which most of the people are unable to bear and they are the worst affected as is evident from the Table 2.1.1. It is also evident that the poorest are the worst affected.

Table 2.1.1: Out of Pocket Expenses and Indebtness

(in US$)

S. No.	*Classification of Out of Pocket Expenses and Indebtness*	*All India*	*Poorest*
1.	Average out of pocket payments made per hospitalisation in government facilities	70	54
2.	Average out of pocket payments made per hospitalisation in private facilities	158	115
3.	Percentage of people indebted due to outpatient care	23	21
4.	Percentage of people indebted due to inpatient care	52	64

Source: Out-of-pocket expenses and indebtness data obtained from National Sample Survey Office (NSSO) 60th round, Government of India (GOI).

The Government of India (GOI) has already made provisions of hospital insurance by subsidiary premium for the poor population. For example, in the year 2003, subsidy of ₹ 100 per family per year was paid to insurance companies for covering the population below poverty line. Universal health insurance scheme spend ₹ 1 for one person, ₹ 1.50 for a household of 5 members and ₹ 2 in respect of 7 members per family per day. This scheme had to be discontinued because it did not get desired response from public.(Economy Watch, 2011). Therefore, in 2008, the Government of India introduced the "Rashtriya Swasthya Bima Yojna" (RSBY). RSBY is uniquely mandated to cover the entire BPL population irrespective of occupational distribution and helps to reduce out-of-pocket expenditure on healthcare and lessen a considerable financial burden on the poor. It has been an important step to supplement the efforts being made to provide quality health care to the poor and under-privileged population. It covers hospitalisation costs up to ₹ 30,000 per annum per household and scheme is jointly funded by the central and state governments in the ratio of 75:25 per cent with a small contribution from the beneficiary household.

SECTION II

2.2 Implementation of Rashtriya Swasthya Bima Yojna in India

RSBY was introduced with a view to providing the BPL households a choice irrespective of access and monitoring risk protection case of indoor treatments. Honourable Prime Minister Manmohan Singh announced this scheme on Gandhi Jayanti in 2007 while registration of beneficiaries started in 2008. The purpose of the scheme is "improving access of BPL families to quality healthcare, hospitalisation and surgery through an identified network of healthcare providers" (RSBY, 2009). By January 2014, 40.13 million families had been enrolled in the scheme and an estimated 140.45 million persons are using the RSBY card. The scheme has been implemented in 536 districts across 30 states and union territories (representing about 83 per cent of the districts in the country). There have been around 7.16 million hospitalisation cases from BPL households availed themselves of the benefits of the scheme. The scheme is on all India bases under which are registered person can get hospitalisation anywhere in India,

By and by the scheme is going to be labourers above poverty line. All types of workers were given the benefit in part or in full measure in the form of subsidy. There is a provision for transport allowance (actual with limit of ₹ 100 per visit) but subject to an annual ceiling of ₹ 1,000; registration fee of ₹ 30 is paid by the household to insurance company per annum; annual premium of ₹ 750 is borne by the Central and State Governments on 75:25, the ratio is 90:10 in the case of the North-Eastern states and Jammu and Kashmir; cost of smart cards also borne by the central government at ₹ 60 per card. It is expected that with the passage of time that number of states and people joining the scheme will increase considerably.

The RSBY is not an health insurance scheme in strict sense as it is a healthcare subsidy scheme. Though there are set guidelines issued by the central government yet there is degree of flexibility in the scheme. States are free to participate in the scheme as per the choices and capabilities. That is the reason this scheme is very popular with most of states who have opted for it quite willingly.

2.2.1 Components of Rashtriya Swasthya Bima Yojna

The activities under the Rashtriya Swasthya Bima Yojna included the following four components:

Component I: Capacity Building and Information Education Communication (CBIEC)

This component is related to that there should be effective roles performed by all the stakeholders for creating the more awareness and penetration among the BPL population across maximum states of the country. The format and structure of the Rashtriya Swasthya Bima Yojna has a need to implement activities which would be further categorised into two periods. During the first period strong co-operation among the central government, state governments and the insurance companies is very required. In this stage proper information regarding the total BPL families of the villages with the planning, management, administration and implementation of enrolling the BPL people and to distribute the smart cards is of great need. The listed of hospitals is occurred at the second stage. The training has given to employees and staff of hospitals to implementing smart card readers, fingerprint scanners and software.

Component II: Management Information System (MIS)

It aimed at effective monitoring of the scheme at the central level. During the initial stages of implementation, effective resources had been used or settlement of enrolling systems and hospital transactions. These systems had been framing for providing the information at back end at the right time.

Component III: Monitoring and Evaluation (M and E)

It deals with producing data and detailed analysis of the scheme of its processes and results. The M and E process under the RSBY involved participation of government counterparts, academics, health officials an evidence-based system of to create rules and policies for outcomes. The M and E process is based on three steps. The first stage is consulting the stakeholders with formation of small groups of workers and employees. Pilotstage is the second one where the M and E activities are work as a guidance to prepare the projects in a reliable, regular and relevant manner. The third stage is implementation where the projects are implemented for a three to five years period.

Component IV: Institutional Development and Project Management (IDPM)

This component make assure that assistance is given to central government and state governments of different states for creation of organisations for the successful implementation and administration of the RSBY.

2.2.2 Institutional Framework of RSBY

Ministry of Labour and Employment (MOLE) co-ordinates the scheme and lays down the policy framework. Office of the Director General–Labour Welfare plays an important role in the execution of the scheme. Making of decisions regarding format of scheme and execution there are of in the hands of MOLE. Figure 2.2.1 displays the institutional framework of RSBY. The scheme is implemented at the state level through a specially created body known as the state nodal agency (SNA).

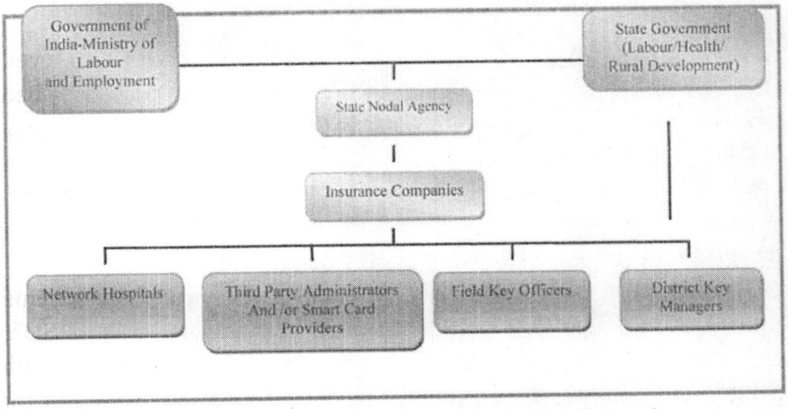

Source: RSBY institutional framework obtained from www.rsby.gov.in.

Figure 2.2.1: RSBY Institutional Framework.

In various departments, there have been constituted SNAs. It is for state government to decide which department for instance Department of Labour, Department of Health and by Department of Rural Development would be serve as SNA in scheme. In most of the state's SNAs a kind of society or trust operates with suitable registration. In some areas the jobs have been assigning to some pre-existing society or trust. The SNA is responsible for supervision and implementation of the scheme and making arrangements with insurance companies as per the guidelines. Insurance companies are selected through bidding to participate in the bid. An insurance company must have a valid licence from the IRDA at the time of application. Fifteen general insurance companies were involved in bidding process for different districts, and 11 general insurance companies were busy by the RSBY out of which four are public general insurance companies while seven are private general insurance providers. In terms of the number of districts served, four of the five leading insurers for RSBY are from the public sector. ICICI Lombard (121 districts) is the only private general insurer in the top five. The insurance companies are responsible for enlisted of hospitals and make sure that their organisational structure meets scheme empanelment criteria. Registration of members is to be done by insurer companies under the supervision of a field key officer nominated by district key manager of the scheme oversees the functioning and supervises the officials under him. District key managers keep a watch on the process of registration of beneficiaries and also monitored and evaluate the execution of the scheme in their jurisdiction.

It is expected of insurance companies to set up a RSBY helpline and call centre in every district. These companies also undertake IEC activities at pre-enrollment stage. After enrollment, IEC becomes primarily the state responsibility. Insurance companies often hire third-party administrators (TPAs) to support beneficiary enrollment, hospital empanellment and claim processing services. The insurers or their TPAs may also hire smart card providers to support the enrollment process and issuing of smart cards. RSBY depends on insurance companies to a very great extent because these act as a middle person in the performance of functions of RSBY. This is due to the fact that SNA's are not able to handle this responsibility. In more states, labour departments act as SNA's and official of the department are not conversant with methods of health system and contracting the mode of hospitals. Most of district key managers hailing from department of labour and qualified for their roles assigned to them under RSBY. To deal with the situation MOLE has to engage some data management agency for the purpose of collection and analysing of data regarding claims and utilisation of services.

2.2.3 Involvement of Public and Private Sector

The RSBY characterises a successful model of symbiotic co-operation between public and private insurance companies. This is the scheme which has something for every stakeholder. Government itself feels the necessity of joining hands with private insurance companies to implement RSBY. The public and private sector players and their roles in the RSBY are shown in Figure 2.2.2.

(a) Central and State Government: RSBY is a scheme of the Government of India. The Ministry of Labour explains the standard rules, plans, procedures, technology, methods for monitoring and evaluation of the scheme across states. The SNA is responsible for implementation of the scheme at the lower level, monitoring of the scheme makes it a unified scheme between the central and state governments. The scheme is financed by both central and the state governments. Seventy-five per cent of contribution by central government in case of premium which is more for North-Eastern states and Jammu and Kashmir to 90 per cent. Rest of the amount is being paid by the concerned states (Gerard and Nagpal, 2012).

In addition to its financing commitment outlined, the Government of India shall undertake the following actions in order to operationalise the Health Insurance scheme:

(a) Issuance and periodic revision of guidelines for the Scheme.

(b) Establishment of an Approval and Monitoring Committee to assess health insurance proposals submitted by State Governments for Government of India financing contribution.

(c) In consultation with the States, development of such protocols and common standards as may be necessary to ensure effective functioning of the Scheme on a national basis. This would include determination of the protocol for nationally unique identification numbers for BPL families, specification of the minimal technical standards of the smart card, ensuring timely transfer of the Central financing share of insurance premia, establishment of common reporting protocols for States as part of Scheme monitoring and such other design and implementation issues considered necessary for the functioning of a coherent national system.

(d) Establishment of a Technical Support Cell within the Ministry of Labour and Employment which would provide expert inputs to Central and State Governments on matters pertaining to the design, implementation and monitoring/evaluation of the Scheme. The Cell would be headed by a Senior Advisor, who would be assisted by two Advisors, database management team, support staff and such other expert personnel as determined from time to time to be necessary to support effective implementation of the Scheme. The Cell would carry out the following functions, *inter alia*:

  (i) Provide technical support to States in development of health insurance schemes for submission to the Central Government.

  (ii) Provide ongoing support to State Governments (co-ordinating with similar Cells at State level) on technical issues in implementation of the Scheme in individual States, including monitoring and evaluation.

(iii) Provide the Approval and Monitoring Committee with such financial estimates as may be necessary to assess the budgetary implications of both Central and State Government commitments under the Scheme.

(iv) Provide technical inputs to the Approval and Monitoring Committee which will allow it to carry out its monitoring and evaluation functions effectively.

(v) Undertake and/or commission detailed evaluation studies on Scheme functioning.

The Responsibilities of the State government are as:

1. Provide certified and validated BPL data as per Planning Commission guidelines and in prescribed format.
2. Designate a Nodal Agency for seamless fund flow (of premiums) to Insurance Co.
3. Designate DKMA for each selected district who then designates FKOs.
4. Help Insurance company prepare enrollment schedule.
5. Help identify locations to hold enrollment camps and facilitate such camps.
6. Help Insurance company to prepare Awareness campaign for beneficiaries.
7. Help Insurance company identify and tie up with hospitals in every district.

(b) Beneficiaries: Beneficiries are the target population for RSBY. According to current estimates, 77.80 million BPL families are there in India and 40.13 million families are enrolled under the scheme (140.45 million BPL People) as on January 2014. Every family can avail the benefits upto five members.The registration fee is ₹ 30 which is to be paid by the beneficiary at annual basis. The new groups which is beyond the below poverty line will be included in the scheme. These include beneficiaries of the National Rural Employment Guarantee Scheme (NREGA), construction workers, postmen on contact basis, railway porters and hawkers, and domestic workers. The Ministry of Labour and Employment has also make clear that RSBY will be open to any person willing to pay the full premium.

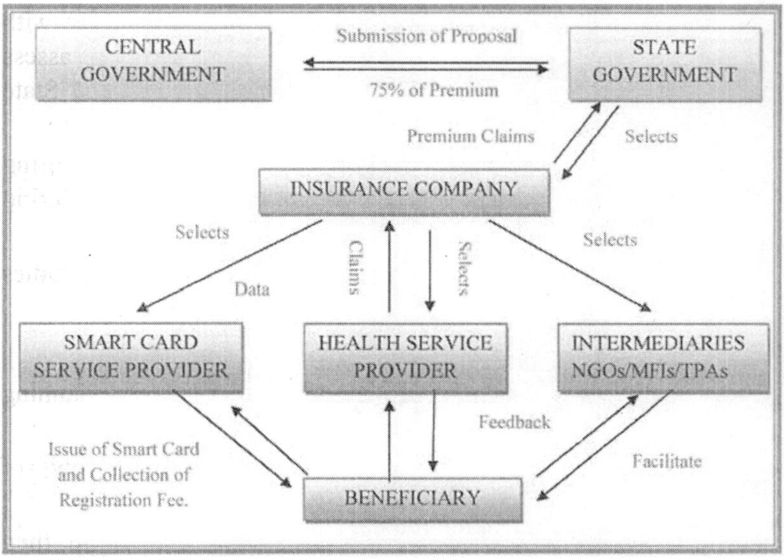

Source: Public Private Partnership Model obtained from Swarup, 2008.

Figure 2.2.2: Public Private Partnership Model of RSBY.

(c) Insurance companies: Insurance companies are the main stakeholders in the implementation of the scheme. Public and government insurance companies can participate as the stakeholder in the system. The roles of the insurance companies are mentioned in the documents of the RSBY as per GOI guidelines. Each state government selects the insurance company through an open tendering process and the company selects by the government according to technical criteria and agrees at lowest insurance premium according to the scheme. The government provides a list of BPL families to insurance companies who are then responsible for enrollment. In order to reach the beneficiaries, insurance companies have to contract. The intermediaries for instance non-governmental organisations (NGOs), micro finance institutions (MFIs) have been contracted for providing information and arranging the awareness camps. The insurance companies are also responsible for the listing of the hospitals. Once smart cards have been distributed to the beneficiaries, the insurance companies are responsible to arrange a kiosk in every village to manage and administer the scheme and there is also a toll-free call centre for the support and guidance of the beneficiaries. The responsibilities of insurance companies are as:

1. Finalise the Smart Card service provider as soon as possible after award of contract.
2. Organise district-level workshops after award of contract.
3. Empanellment of Hospitals as per defined criteria (may take help of State Nodal Agency) and provide a list to the State Government.
4. Prepare brochures to be provided to Beneficiaries along with the RSBY cards at enrollment camps.
5. Monitoring of Enrollment camps.
6. Ensuring provision of devices at the hospitals.
7. Timely Settling claims of the Hospitals.
8. Setting up and maintaining a helpline in each district.
9. Set up and Maintain district kiosks.

(d) Smart Card Service Provider: Smart card is central to the RSBY, as it is a helpful tool in doing the cashless transaction and portability services can also availed throughout India. It would also helpful in the biometric identification of the household. The smart cards distributed to the beneficiaries by the smart card service provider. The ownership of the card are only with the Central Government for

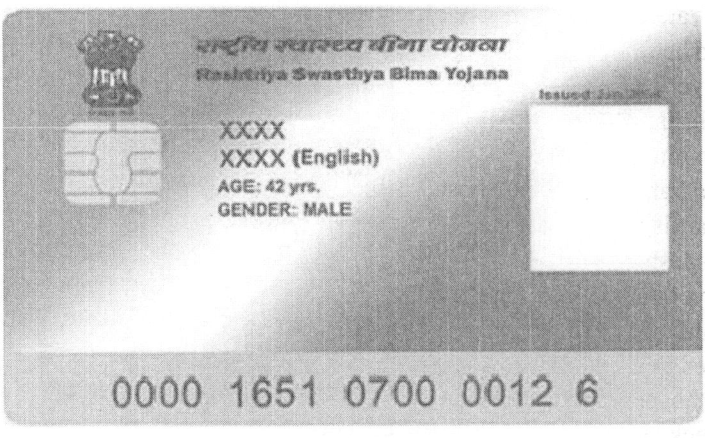

Source: Sample of smart card obtained from www.rsby.gov.in.

Figure 2.2.3: A Sample of Smart Card.

its use in following years. The card is to be given to the household on the spot. The smart card cannot be given to any other or in the absence of head of the family. The photograph is also on the card. The details of the rest of the family members can be added at the district kiosk which has to be maintained by the insurance companies.

The responsibilities of service providers are as:

1. At the district-level workshop
   (a) Demonstrate and explain solution to District officials and Village functionaries
   (b) Issue IA cards to 1stset of FKOS
   (c) Train FKOs on use of IA cards.
2. Conduct enrollment as per route chart and issue cards on the spot.
3. Collect ₹ 30 fee from Beneficiary and handover card on the spot.
4. Installing h/w used for smart card operations in Hospitals and train them on usage.
5. Prepare and get the transaction s/w certified.
6. Deployment of s/w that can compile and transmit data electronically to the state nodal agency.

(e) Network Provider- Hospitals: Beneficiaries can avail hospitalisation facilities through any of the 11,565 empanelled hospitals spread across 536 districts as on January 2014, of which 7,328 are private and 4,237 are public hospitals with 63:37 providing choice and better access to beneficiaries.[1] The share of public hospitals network is very high in Rajasthan, Himachal Pradesh, Kerala, Uttrakhand, Odisha, Assam, Tripura, Meghalaya, Mizoram, Arunachal Pradesh, Jammu and Kashmir and Andhra Pradesh.The opposite is the case of Gujarat, Bihar, Uttar Pradesh, Punjab, West Bengal, Haryana, Nagaland, Chattisgarh, Karnataka, Manipur, Puducherry, Delhi and Madhya Pradesh.This probably reflects the working relationship of the state government department that supervises the scheme in each of these states. The same process is to be followed that when a beneficiary goes to empanelled hospital, a designated RSBY helpdesk, arranged by hospital staff comes into consideration. The helpdesk registers and check the validity of the beneficiary's details, using the smart card with patient's thumbprint. If the hospitalisation is required to the beneficiary the hospital make sure of the packages and the availability of funds. If the required service is not according to the pre-defined packages, a approval is must and the helpdesk consults with the insurer to make sure the amount paid to the hospital. On completion of the treatment, the amount is minus from the insured amount in the card. The hospital also sends this information electronically to the insurance company or TPA for reimbursement of the claim. Claims must be paid within the time limit agreed upon in the contract between the insurer and the network hospital in 21 days.

(f) Intermediaries: The main intermediaries are theTPAs and NGOs which are assisting in create awareness camps. There are 29 active third party administrators (TPAs) in India. TPAs are required to issue fingerprint scanners, smart card providers at the camps with a time limit of one year. Only those household members who are present at the camp can be enrolled. Frauds can be minimised with these camps because the smart cards provided to only the present households.

2.2.4. Process Flow in RSBY

One of the strengths of RSBY is its well-defined processes including clearly earmarked roles. This section provides an outline of the most important processes of the scheme. It is important to note here that many a times a stakeholder can be outsourced for more than one of its functions.

The broad process flow for RSBY is as follows:

1. Setting up of State Nodal Agency
   - (i) Once the decision to implement RSBY is taken by a state government, an independent body called the 'State Nodal Agency' or SNA is set up.
   - (ii) The agency is staffed with government employees and professionals. It generates its revenue through a registration fee of ₹ 30 per year per family paid by the beneficiaries.
2. Preparation of Beneficiary Data
   - (i) An SNA collects/prepares beneficiary data in the specified RSBY format.

(ii) Data for different categories is collected from different sources and merged generally into one dataset.

3. Validation of Beneficiary Data and Generation of Unique Relationship Number (URN)

   (i) Beneficiary data is sent by SNA to Ministry of Labour and Employment. The team at MOLE validates that this data is in the specified format.

   (ii) URN, which is unique across the country, is generated for each beneficiary family, and the data is encrypted so that only an appointed agency can decrypt it.

   (iii) This data is then uploaded on the RSBY website by the MOLE.

4. Selection of Insurance Company

   (i) An insurance company is selected by an SNA through an open-bidding process.

   (ii) An insurance company can be selected for one or more districts, however, for one district only one insurance company can be selected.

5. Empanellment of Healthcare Providers

   (i) Based on the list of healthcare providers given by the SNA/district administration, the insurance company empanells the healthcare providers who fulfill the empanellment criteria.

   (ii) Necessary hardware and software are installed in the hospitals so as to facilitate transaction at the hospital electronically. Private hospitals have to pay for the hardware cost, while for public hospitals the cost is paid by the insurance companies.

   (iii) Hospital representatives are trained by the insurance companies to use the software and hardware.

6. Enrollment of Beneficiaries

   (i) An electronic list of eligible beneficiary families is provided to insurers by the SNA through the RSBY website.

   (ii) An enrollment schedule for each village, along with dates, is prepared by the insurance company with the help of district and block officials. An insurance company is provided a maximum of four months to enrol beneficiary families in each district.

(iii) Insurance companies hire intermediaries to reach out to the beneficiaries before the enrollment. In addition, the beneficiary list is posted in each village at the enrollment station and prominent places prior to the enrollment camp. The date/location of the enrollment camp are also publicised in advance.

(iv) Moving enrollment stations are established at local centres (e.g., panchayat office) at each village at least once a year. These stations are equipped by the insurer with the hardware to collect fingerprints and photographs of the members of the families covered and a printer to print smart cards with photo.

(v) A local government official (field key-officer or FKO) is mandated to be present at the enrollment centres and he/she inserts his/her own government-issued smart card and provide his/her fingerprint to verify the legitimacy of the enrollment for each family. Data of each beneficiary family verified by the FKOs is also stored in the card of the FKOs. This way, each enrolee can be tracked to a particular official.

(vi) The smart card, along with an information packet describing benefits, hospitals in network, etc. is provided to all enrolees once they have paid the ₹ 30 registration fees. The process normally takes less than 10 minutes.

(vii) At the end of the enrollment camp, details of all the enrolled households is sent to the district authority and the SNA by the insurer. The list of enrolled households is maintained centrally.

7. Payment of Premium

(i) Based on the number of families enrolled, the insurance company is paid a premium. This number is calculated based on the data downloaded from the FKO card and encrypted data generated by the software.

(ii) This premium is shared between the state and the central governments. After the payment is made by the state, the central government releases its share.

8. Utilisation of Services

(i) A beneficiary, after receiving the smart card and after the commencement of the insurance policy, can visit any empanelled hospitals across the country to receive cashless treatment.

(ii) The process of getting the benefits at the hospital is a paperless one and no documents need to be shown to get the benefit. The fingerprint of the beneficiary is matched with the fingerprint stored in the smart card and once it matches the beneficiary receives the treatment at the hospital.

(iii) The hospitals send online data at each stage of admission of the beneficiary to the government and the insurance company. After the patient is discharged, the hospital sends the claims data to the insurance company and the state and central governments. After due diligence, the insurance company settles the claims of the hospitals, which is done online. Hospitals also need not provide any paper for the claim process.

2.2.5. Use of Technology in RSBY

The use of technology in RSBY is one of the highlights of the scheme. It is perhaps one of the few schemes in the developing world where technology has been leveraged at this scale for delivering social sector benefits.

RSBY uses different types of technologies at various stages. Each type of technology is there for a different purpose. The following technologies are being used in the scheme:

1. Smart Card Technology- A smart card is given to each beneficiary family at the time of enrollment in the scheme. The smart card, which contains fingerprint and photograph, is prepared and printed on the spot in the village by the insurer and handed over to the beneficiary.

2. Biometric Technology- Fingerprints of all the beneficiaries are collected on the spot. A thumb impression of each of the beneficiary is stored in the smart card. This fingerprint is used to verify the identity of the beneficiaries at the hospitals. Biometric verification is also done by a government officer to authenticate the identity of the beneficiary for enrollment in the scheme.

3. Key Management System- The key management system helps in higher security, reduces frauds and at the same time improves accountability. The FKO needs to be present at the enrollment station and his/her role is to verify each beneficiary family using his/her own smart card and fingerprints. This ensures that a correct beneficiary is issued the card by the insurer. Similarly, this type of security smart card is provided at the empanelled hospitals and the district kiosk (lost or damaged card can be issued and modifications in the card can be done at the district kiosk).The only persons who have authorised security smart cards can access the chip of the beneficiary smart card for any transaction/modification.

4. Web-based Data Transfer- RSBY has been able to position itself as a paperless scheme with the help of technology. Claims are submitted online by the hospitals and similarly insurer can make online payments to the hospitals. In addition to this, a robust back-end data management system has been developed for RSBY which ensures smooth flow of real time data from across India to the state and the central governments.

5. Web Portal Services- The web portal of RSBY has multiple roles. It not only provides the details of RSBY with the outside world, but also acts as the portal for data transfer, data sharing and a monitoring tool for the internal stakeholders of the scheme. The aim of the scheme is to use technology not only for control of fraud and monitoring, but also to find innovative solutions. For example, the enrollment software has been designed in a way that if the spouse is part of the BPL list, then the software makes it compulsory to insure her as well.

The smart card has huge potential to deliver other social security schemes through the same IT platform to the same set of beneficiaries. This can bring down the cost and improve transparency.

Especially schemes that are targeted at the same set of beneficiaries can be delivered through the same smart card platform in an efficient way.

2.2.6. Use of RSBY Technology Platform to Deliver Other Social Security Schemes

RSBY provides a smart card-based technology platform that has the potential to deliver for many other social security schemes. Many social security schemes are being run for the same target segment by the various ministries of the government and at present separate efforts are being made to reach the same beneficiary for these schemes. RSBY provides an opportunity to deliver various schemes to the same beneficiary at the same time. The Government of Chhattisgarh took a decision to use RSBY smart card for delivering food subsidy through PDS. Entitlement of PDS is loaded in the RSBY smart card, and the beneficiaries can visit any empanelled fair price shop for their entitled foodgrains, kerosene, etc. after biometric verification. Data regarding purchase flow daily to the government server and government can track this on a daily basis. Experience from this experiment has resulted in substantial savings for the state government and also at the same time it has empowered the beneficiaries. The Government of Punjab has experimented by delivering the life and disability insurance scheme called the Aam Aadmi Bima Yojna (AABY) through the RSBY smart card platform in one district. A beneficiary is enrolled at the same time for both RSBY and AABY. This makes not only the process of enrolling in these schemes easier, but also reduces distribution cost. Such experiments show the potential of RSBY card that it can be used for delivering many social security benefits to the same beneficiary families.

2.2.7 Strengths and Weaknesses of RSBY

1. **Significant Financial Protection and Reduction in Out of Pocket Expenditure:** Through this scheme, the government has been able to provide cashless medical services to needy people, who would not otherwise have been able to afford the service.
2. **An Economical Model:** By fixing package prices, RSBY has made a major conceptual advance on existing healthcare delivery models. The concept of package prices for an

indicative length of stay makes healthcare costs transparent and this imposes a natural check on prices. The average cost per treatment is around ₹ 4000. Premium remains on an average ₹ 500 per family per annum.

3. **Encouraging Better Maintenance of Patient Records:**The NLI report said that as many as 86 per cent patients were provided a discharge summary. Records of treatment are very important to maintain continuity of care and this is one of the most important areas that need attention in healthcare in India today.

Observed Weaknesses of RSBY

1. **Little or No Involvement of SNA:** The SNA being the backbone of the scheme at the States lacks adequate capacity to monitor the activities within the scheme. Another cascading issue is that of the performance data, which is not provided by the Insurance Company to the SNA, which leaves the SNA with no scope for any further action.
2. **Involvement of TPA in Operating the Scheme at States:** The TPA's are employed by the Insurance Companies to process the claims raised by the hospitals and other administrative tasks. It has also been observed that in some States, the TPA's are also conducting enrollments on behalf of the Insurance Company. The Committee has also observed that TPA's in some states have sub-contracted their responsibilities to other agencies unknown to the SNA. This has diluted the focus of the Insurance Company towards providing the benefits of the scheme to the end beneficiary.
3. **Evolving Concept of Re-Insurance in RSBY:** It has been observed that Insurance Companies associated with RSBY are passing their risk to Re-insurers. The Re-insurers are paid an amount to cover the risk for the RSBY insurer, which leads to low claim ratio at the States.
4. **Low Level of Awareness About RSBY:** Despite the scheme being managed from the State, the awareness of the benefits of the scheme are not known to many beneficiaries. This has also contributed to the low utilisation of the scheme. Though the responsibility of creating awareness of the scheme lies

with the Insurance Company, the utilisation data does not depict awareness of the scheme. Additionally, the SNA who could have played a key role in increasing awareness of the scheme lacked the institutional support and the capacity.

6. **Dissatisfaction in the States:** There has been dissatisfaction expressed by a few state governments regarding the structure of the scheme, from time to time. Three major state governments, Tamil Nadu, Maharashtra and Andhra Pradesh have refused to participate in the scheme and have preferred to run their own state government-funded health insurance schemes. Other governments have flagged issues about the implementation methodology adopted in the scheme. Excessive authority given to Insurance companies and poor monitoring methodology are among the chief complaints.
7. **No Clinical Pathways in the Scheme:** A scheme which intends to provide good healthcare to people, should have some clinical pathways for the various procedures especially in view of the fact that services are being purchased from private sector hospitals. However, this has not been the case so far. This could be one reason why the quality of services provided remains quite variable.
8. **Reports of Fraud and Medical Malpractice:** A report by Amicus Advisory and several media reports have flagged the issue of large number of ghost cards. There are also cases of suspect procedures being performed needlessly although without treatment protocols, there is no way of judge if there is any truth in the charges.
9. **Perverse Financial Incentives:** One of the major problems reported has been that while the scheme incentivises hospital treatment to patients, it has no incentives for medical management since OPD costs are not covered. Many evaluations have reported high use of surgical packages.

Due to a great deal of dissatisfaction among state governments, the government felt a need to study the experiences of various state governments providing health coverage to people and on the basis of these inputs, to look at revamping the RSBY, adopt best practices and to address the weaknesses reported.

2.2.8 Enrollment of BPL Households under RSBY in India

Table 2.2.1 shows implementation status of Rashtriya Swasthya Bima Yojna in various states of India. The programme was monitored by Ministry of Labour and Employment at the Government of India, with the nodal department in each state. From a humble beginning in the year 2008, with only two states implementing RSBY, whereas, by the end of 2008, eleven states have enrolled under RSBY scheme, eleven more states enrolled in 2009 and by the end of 2010, four more states enrolled for Rashtriya Swasthya Bima Yojna and till January, 2014, total 30 states/ UTs had enrolled with Rashtriya Swasthya Bima Yojna Scheme.

The total BPL families in India were 77.80 millions, out of which 40.13 million (51.6 per cent) had enrolled with RSBY scheme up to January, 2014, about 35 million cards (covering 122.5 million persons) were issued under the scheme. There were 645 districts in thirty states/ UTs and 536 districts enrolled for RSBY scheme out of which in 468 districts, enrollment had been completed and was in progress in 38 districts. The take-up ratio showed the coverage of the scheme and the maximum take-up ratio of 84.8 per cent was of Kerala followed by 74.6 per cent in Andhra Pradesh and 71.6 per cent in Himachal Pradesh. The take up ratios of Rajasthan, Chandigarh, Odisha, Tripura and Puducherry were in the range of 60-70 per cent. The take-up ratios of Bihar, Assam, Manipur, Jammu and Kashmir and Maharashtra were in the range of 50-60 per cent. The take up ratio of Gujarat, Uttar Pradesh, Jharkhand, Uttrakhand, Punjab, Haryana, Nagaland, Chattisgarh, Meghalaya, Mizoram, Karnataka, Arunachal Pradesh and Manipur were in the range of 30-50 per cent. The minimum take up ratio 9.6 per cent was of Delhi.

The above analysis bespeaks of success of implementation of RSBY scheme with maximum BPL families having enrolled for it. With more categories being added to the scheme and more states joining in, this number is expected to grow further in the future.

2.2.9 Percentage of Participation, Enrollment and Coverage of States

From the Table 2.2.2, it is found that more than 90 per cent of districts participated in RSBY were in twenty two states viz. Gujarat, Bihar, Himachal Pradesh, Kerala, Uttar Pradesh, Maharashtra,

Table 2.2.1: Enrollment of Below Poverty Line Households under Rashtriya Swasthya Bima Yojna in India

Sr. No.	States/UTs	Date of Enrollment	Number of Districts						BPL Families		
			Total Districts	Selected Districts	Enrollment Completed in Districts	Enrollment In Progress in Districts	Percentage of Participation of Districts	Percentage of Enrollment Complete in Districts	BPL Families in Selected Districts	BPL Families Enrolled	Take-up Ratio
1.	Rajasthan	27.02.08	33	33	6	26	100	18	36,85,055	25,83,767	70.1
2.	Gujarat	18.08.08	27	26	26	-	96	100	43,70,200	17,90,585	41.0
3.	Bihar	20.08.08	38	38	38	-	100	100	1,20,18,876	65,72,928	54.7
4.	Tamil Nadu	19.09.08	32	2	2	-	6	100	N.A.	N.A.	N.A.
5.	Himachal Pradesh	1.10.08	12	12	12	-	100	100	5,54,693	3,96,938	71.6
6.	Kerala	2.10.08	14	14	14	-	100	100	34,46,235	29,20,857	84.8
7.	Maharashtra	2.10.08	35	32	32	.	91	100	45,09,135	22,64,138	50.2
8.	Uttar Pradesh	3.10.08	75	75	75	-	100	100	1,10,60,686	46,53,382	42.1
9.	Jharkhand	21.10.08	24	24	24	-	100	100	33,34,364	16,29,139	48.9
10.	Uttrakhand	1.12.08	13	13	13	-	100	100	7,46,197	2,85,435	38.3
11.	Punjab	16.12.08	22	22	22	-	100	100	4,53,936	1,58,517	34.9
12.	West Bengal	1.1.09	19	19	19	-	100	100	96,38,922	54,24,761	56.3
13.	Haryana	13.02.09	21	21	21	-	100	100	12,63,813	4,52,045	35.8
14.	Nagaland	25.02.09	11	11	9	2	100	82	4,23,886	1,38,904	32.8
15.	Chandigarh (U.T.)	28.02.09	1	1	1	-	100	100	9,548	5,854	61.3
16.	Goa	13.03.09	2	2	2	-	100	100	N.A.	N.A.	N.A.
17.	Chhattisgarh	10.06.09	27	27	27	-	100	100	59,64,645	28,82,329	48.3
18.	Delhi	01.07.09	10	10	1	-	100	10	9,87,824	95,597	9.6
19.	Odisha	10.09.09	30	30	30	-	100	100	57,73,709	36,01,602	62.4
20.	Assam	11.10.09	27	23	17	3	85	74	25,87,583	13,35,982	51.6
21.	Tripura	12.11.09	7	7	7	-	100	100	7,86,913	5,05,327	64.2
22.	Meghalaya	11.12.09	11	11	11	-	100	100	4,86,695	1,99,065	40.9
23.	Karnataka	08.02.10	30	30	30	-	100	100	40,76,642	16,76,249	41.1

(Cond...)

24.	Mizoram	13.08.10	8	8	8	-	100	100	2,21,814	1,03,545	46.7
25.	Manipur	23.09.10	9	6	5	1	67	83	1,20,237	57,995	48.2
26.	Arunachal Pradesh	02.11.10	16	14	10	-	88	71	90,312	39,615	43.8
27.	Jammu and Kashmir	16.12.11	15	14	2	-	93	14	66,005	35,521	53.8
28.	Puducherry	21.06.12	4	1	1	-	25	100	15,142	9,486	62.6
29.	Andhra Pradesh	3.11.12	23	1	1	-	4	100	2,759	2,060	74.6
30.	Madhya Pradesh	7.11.12	50	9	2	6	18	22	11,10,545	3,18,314	28.7
	Total		**645**	**536**	**468**	**38**	**83**	**87**	**7,78,06,371**	**4,01,39,937**	**51.6**

Source: Author's calculation.

Note: Take up ratio and percentages computed from data obtained from www.rsby.gov.in, as on 17th January 2014.

Note: Take up ratio is the ratio of BPL families enrolled to BPL families in selected districts.

N.A.: Data not available.

Uttrakhand, Punjab, West Bengal, Haryana, Rajasthan, Chandigarh, Goa, Chhattisgarh, Delhi, Tripura, Mizoram, Jharkhand, Odisha, Meghalaya, Karnataka and Jammu and Kashmir. Arunachal Pradesh, Nagaland and Assam were three states whose participation of districts was in the range of 70-90 per cent and Manipur was the only state whose districts participation was in the range of 50-70 per cent.

It was found that less than 50 per cent of districts of four states viz. Tamil Nadu, Andhra Pradesh, Puducherry and Madhya Pradesh had completed the enrollment and not even a single district was in the range of 50-70 per cent. More than 90 per cent enrollment process had been completed in selected districts of twenty two states viz. Tamil Nadu, Himachal Pradesh, Kerala, Chandigarh, Goa, Puducherry, Odisha, Karnataka, Uttrakhand, Mizoram, Tripura, Meghalaya, Gujarat, Bihar, Maharashtra, Chhattisgarh, Punjab, Jharkhand, Uttar Pradesh, West Bengal, Haryana and Andhra Pradesh.

The districts enrolled in the range of 71-90 per cent were in four states viz. Manipur, Nagaland, Assam and Arunachal Pradesh. Four states viz. Delhi, Rajasthan, Jammu and Kashmir and Madhya Pradesh had completed less than 50 per cent of enrollment. As far as coverage of BPL families was concerned, the table also illustrated that not even a single state had covered more than 90 per cent BPL families.

The percentages of BPL families covered in the range of 71-90 per cent were in four states viz. Kerala, Rajasthan, Andhra Pradesh and Himachal Pradesh. Nine states participated within the range of 50-70 per cent were West Bengal, Chandigarh, Odisha, Bihar, Tripura, Assam, Maharashtra, Jammu and Kashmir and Puducherry. Less than 50 per cent of BPL families were covered in seventeen states viz. Uttar Pradesh, Punjab, Haryana, Delhi, Mizoram, Gujarat, Tamil Nadu, Jharkhand, Uttrakhand, Nagaland, Goa, Meghalaya, Chhattisgarh, Karnataka, Manipur, Madhya Pradesh and Arunachal Pradesh.

Table 2.2.2: Percentage of Participation, Enrollment and Coverage of States

Percentage of Participation of Districts in States/UTs		
No. of States/UTs	*States/UTs*	*Percentage of Districts*
22	Gujarat, Bihar, H.P., Kerala, U.P., Maharashtra, Uttrakhand, Punjab, West Bengal, Haryana, Rajasthan, Chandigarh, Goa, Chhattisgarh, Delhi, Tripura, Mizoram, Jharkhand, Odisha, Meghalaya, Karnataka, Jammu and Kashmir	>90
3	Arunachal Pradesh, Nagaland, Assam	71-90
1	Manipur	50-70
4	Tamil Nadu, Andhra Pradesh, Puducherry, Madhya Pradesh	<50
Percentage of Enrollment Completed in Districts in States/UTs		
No. of States/UTs	*States/UTs*	*Percentage of Districts*
22	Tamil Nadu, Himachal Pradesh, Kerala, Chandigarh, Goa, Puducherry, Odisha, Karnataka, Uttrakhand, Mizoram, Tripura, Meghalaya, Gujarat, Bihar, Maharashtra, Chhattisgarh, Punjab, Jharkhand, Uttar Pradesh, West Bengal, Haryana, Andhra Pradesh	>90
4	Manipur, Arunachal Pradesh, Nagaland, Assam	71-90
4	Delhi, Jammu and Kashmir, Madhya Pradesh and Rajasthan	<50
Percentage of BPL Families Covered in Districts in States/UTs		
No. of States/UTs	*States/UTs*	*Percentage of Districts*
4	Kerala, Himachal Pradesh, Rajasthan, Andhra Pradesh	71-90
9	West Bengal, Chandigarh, Odisha, Bihar, Tripura, Assam, Maharashtra, Jammu and Kashmir and Puducherry.	50-70
17	Uttar Pradesh, Punjab, Haryana, Delhi, Mizoram, Gujarat, Tamil Nadu, Jharkhand, Uttrakhand, Nagaland, Goa, Madhya Pradesh, Meghalaya, Chhattisgarh, Manipur, Karnataka and Arunachal Pradesh	<50

Source: Author's calculation.

Note: Percentages of participation, enrollment and coverage of states computed from data obtained from www.rsby.gov.in, as on 17 January, 2014.

2.2.10 Empanellment of Hospitals

Table 2.2.3 shows empanellment of healthcare providers and the total healthcare providers in RSBY were 11,565 out of which 7,328 were private and 4,237 were public hospitals. The maximum hospitals were in Uttar Pradesh i.e., 1,984 out of which 63.2 per cent were private hospitals and 36.8 per cent were public. Gujarat was the second leading state in which total hospitals were 1,424 out of which 65.8 per cent were private and 34.2 per cent were public hospitals

It was found that Arunachal Pradesh had 100 per cent share of public hospitals and 98 per cent, 95 per cent and 84 per cent were the share of public hospitals in Tripura, Meghalaya and Mizoram respectively. The share of public hospital network was very high in case of Himachal Pradesh, Chhattisgarh, Assam, Uttrakhand and Odisha. The opposite was the case of Punjab, Uttar Pradesh, Karnataka, Madhya Pradesh, Haryana, Nagaland and West Bengal, Delhi, Manipur, Puducherry had 100 per cent share and Maharashtra had 99 per cent share of private hospitals.There was not any hospital empanelled in Tamil Nadu and Goa.The maximum BPL families 19,843 have enrolled per hospital were in Nagaland as there were 86 per cent public hospitals and 14 per cent private hospitals followed by Manipur which enrolled 9,665 BPL families.The minimum BPL families 294 enrolled per hospital were in Arunachal Pradesh with ratio of 43 per cent and 57 per cent hospitals followed by 472 BPL families enrolled per hospital were in Punjab with ratio of 52 per cent private and 48 per cent public hospitals which further followed by 732 BPL families enrolled per hospital of Chandigarh with the ratio of 50:50 in case of public and private hospitals.

Figure 2.2.4 depicts the share of public and private hospitals under RSBY scheme in various states of India. The share of private hospitals was maximum in comparison to public hospitals in 14 states viz. Gujarat, Bihar, Uttar Pradesh, Punjab, West Bengal, Haryana, Nagaland, Chhattisgarh, Karnataka, Manipur, Puducherry, Maharashtra, Delhi and Madhya Pradesh. The opposite was in the case of 12 states viz. Rajasthan, Himachal Pradesh, Kerala, Uttrakhand, Odisha, Assam, Tripura, Meghalaya, Mizoram, Arunachal Pradesh, Jammu and Kashmir and Andhra Pradesh. The share of private and public hospitals

Table 2.2.3: Healthcare Empanellment of Hospitals in RSBY

S. No.	States/UTs	Selected Districts	No. of Private Hospitals	No. of Public Hospitals	No. of Total Hospitals	Share of Private Hospitals (in Percentage)	Share of Public Hospitals (in percentage)	BPL Families Enrolled	No. of BPL Families Enrolled per Hospital
1.	Rajasthan	33	229	453	682	34	66	25,83,767	3,788
2.	Gujarat	26	937	487	1,424	66	34	17,90,585	1,257
3.	Bihar	38	865	100	965	90	10	65,72,928	6,811
4.	Tamil Nadu	2	N.A.	N.A.	N.A.	N.A.	N.A.	N.A.	N.A.
5.	Himachal Pradesh	12	23	171	194	12	88	3,96,938	2,046
6.	Kerala	14	146	161	307	48	52	29,20,857	9,514
7.	Maharashtra	32	1,207	15	1,222	99	1	22,64,138	1,853
8.	Uttar Pradesh	75	1,254	730	1,984	63	37	46,53,382	2,346
9.	Jharkhand	24	217	220	437	50	50	16,29,139	3,728
10.	Uttrakhand	13	49	94	143	34	66	2,85,435	1,996
11.	Punjab	22	175	161	336	52	48	1,58,517	472
12.	West Bengal	19	568	65	633	90	10	54,24,761	8,570
13.	Haryana	21	429	33	462	93	7	4,52,045	978
14.	Nagaland	11	6	1	7	86	14	1,38,904	19,843
15.	Chandigarh	1	4	4	8	50	50	5,854	732
16.	Goa	2	N.A.	N.A.	N.A.	N.A.	N.A.	N.A.	N.A.
17.	Chhattisgarh	27	349	279	628	56	44	28,82,329	4,590
18.	Delhi	10	35	N.A.	35	100	N.A.	95,597	2731
19.	Odisha	30	137	408	545	25	75	36,01,602	6,608
20.	Assam	23	32	134	166	19	81	13,35,982	8,048
21.	Tripura	7	1	53	54	2	98	5,05,327	9,358

(Cond...)

22.	Meghalaya	11	10	188	198	5	95	1,99,065	1,005
23.	Karnataka	30	546	328	874	63	37	16,76,249	1,918
24.	Mizoram	8	15	78	93	16	84	1,03,545	1,113
25.	Manipur	6	6	-	6	100	-	57,995	9,665
26.	Arunachal Pradesh	14	-	11	11	-	100	39,615	3,601
27.	Jammu and Kashmir	14	5	15	20	25	75	35,521	1,776
28.	Puducherry	1	4	-	4	100	-	9,486	2,372
29.	Andhra Pradesh	1	3	4	7	43	57	2,060	294
30.	Madhya Pradesh	9	76	44	120	63	37	3,18,314	2,653
	Total	**536**	**7,328**	**4,237**	**11,565**	**63.2**	**36.8**	**4,01,39,937**	**3,471**

Source: Author's calculation.

Note: Share of public and private hospitals data obtained from www.rsby.gov.in as on January, 2014.

Note: Number of BPL families enrolled per hospital= BPL families enrolled/Total number of hospitals.

N.A.: Data not available.

were in the ratio of 50:50 in Jharkhand and Chandigarh. Hundred per cent share of private hospitals were found in case of Delhi, Manipur and Puducherry. Arunachal Pradesh was the only state having 100 per cent share of public hospitals. It was found that share of private hospitals was maximum but public hospitals were also empanelled in large number with Rashtriya Swasthya Bima Yojna.

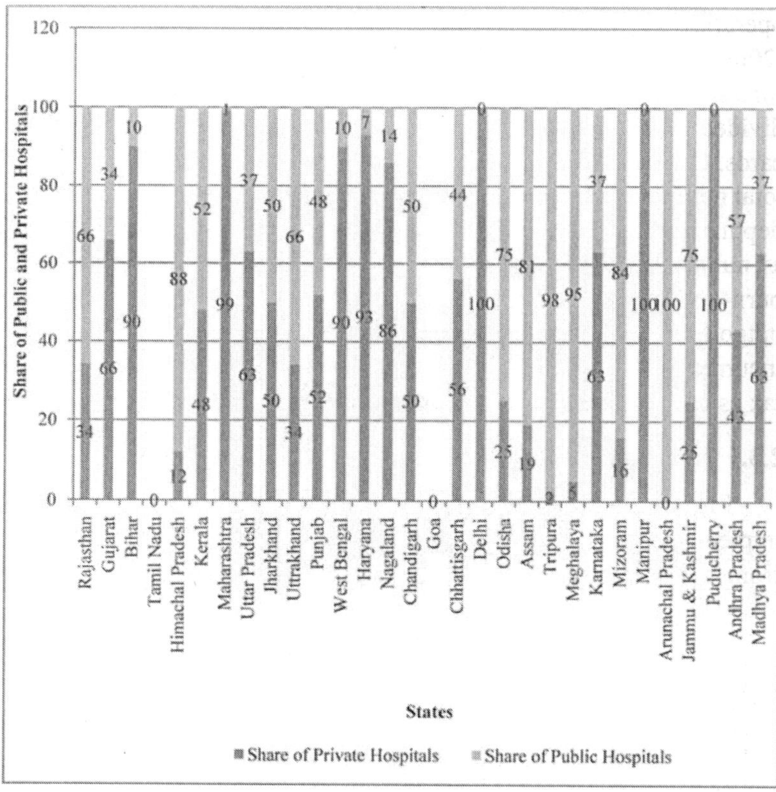

(in Percentage)

Source: Author's self-construction.

Note: Empanellment of public and private hospitals data obtained from www.rsby.gov.in.

Figure 2.2.4: State-wise Number of Private and Public Hospitals Empanelled.

SECTION III

2.3 State-wise Impact of RSBY on BPL Population in India

This section focuses on four key performance indicators (KPIs) – Claims Ratio (utilisation by beneficiaries), Conversion Ratio (a tool for measuring outreach), Hospitalisation Ratio (an indicator of utilisation of healthcare) and Total Expense Ratio (a parameter to judge profit to the insurance company). These key performance indicators were analysed from aggregated state-wise data for the first year of operations (2008-09) for 24 states (314 districts), for the second year (2009-10) for 17 states (182 districts) and for the third year (2010-11) for 5 states (36 districts). Claim Ratio is defined as claim paid to hospital divided by premium paid to insurance company minus cost of smart cards. Conversion ratio i.e., ratio of number of households enrolled to total number of eligible BPL families per district is an indicator of the depth of outreach of the scheme. Hospitalisation ratio which is defined as number of hospitalisation cases divided by total enrollment. The burn-out ratio (evolved specifically for the schemes) determines the outgo from insurance company in terms of percentage of expenditure incurred in payments made to the hospitals, smart card cost and service tax as against the total premium received.

2.3.1 Premium Trends, Smart Cards and Average Family Size

Figure 2.3.1 shows that the districts which have started implementation of RSBY in 2008, the average premium have decreased from ₹ 607 during Round 1 to ₹ 518 in Round ₹ 3.

(in ₹)

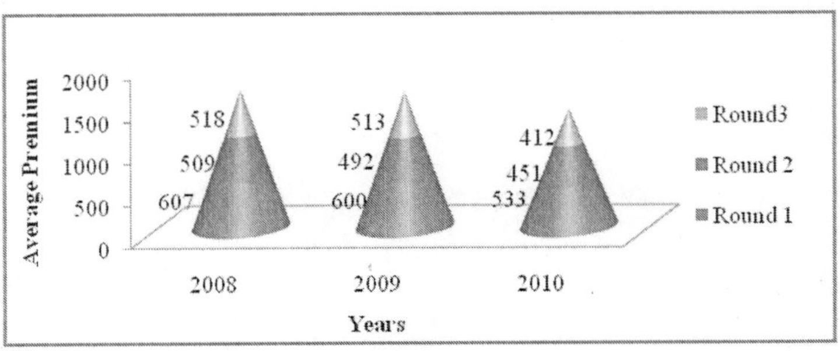

Source: Author's self-construction.

Note: Premium trends data obtained from www.rsby.gov.in.

Figure 2.3.1: Premium Trends in RSBY.

In year 2009, the average premium for fresh districts was ₹ 600 in round 1 which decreased to ₹ 513 in round 3. In year 2010, the average premium for fresh districts was ₹ 533 which decreased to ₹ 412 in round 3. This could be attributed to price correction over the years on the basis of utilisation data, of economies of scale, increase in number of beneficiaries i.e., outreach of the scheme, decrease in cost of smart cards, installation of hardware etc.

Figure 2.3.2 shows the distribution of smart cards and hospitalisation cases. It was found that RSBY commenced on 1st of April 2008 with 4.0 million smart card beneficiaries, over a period of time from the years 2008-09 to 2011-12, the smart card beneficiaries increased from 4.0 million in the year 2008-09 to 13.8 million in year 2009-10 and further increased to 23.3 million in year 2010-11 and 27.9 million in year 2011-12.

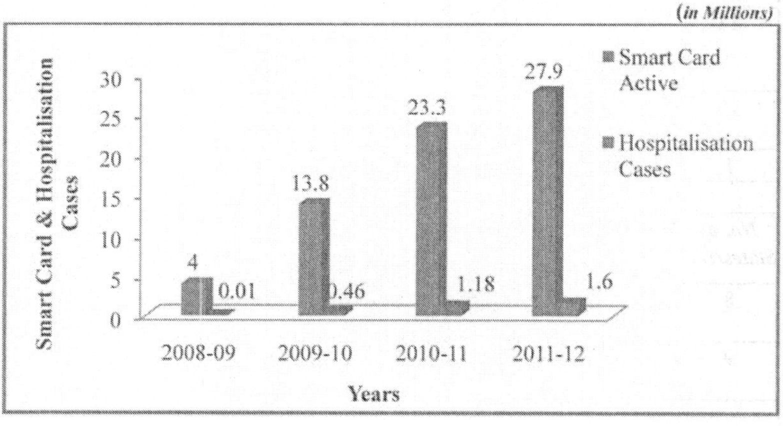

Source: Author's self-construction.

Note: Smart cards and hospitalisation cases data obtained from www.rsby.gov.in.

Figure 2.3.2: Distribution of Smart Cards and Hospitalisation Cases.

In case of hospitalisation cases, these increased from 0.01 to 0.46, 0.46 to 1.18 and 1.18 to 1.6 from years 2008-09 to 2009-10, 2009-10 to 2010-11 and 2011-2012 respectively. The RSBY has influenced and changed the lives of BPL beneficiaries and proved itself as a flagship health insurance scheme in India.

The average family size of round 1, 2 and 3 in various states of India are as shown in the Table 2.3.1. It was found that in round 1, the average family size ranged between greater than two members but less than three members was in Bihar, Haryana, Karnataka, Kerala, Maharashtra, Meghalaya, Odisha, Punjab, Tripura, Uttar Pradesh, Uttrakhand, Goa, Tamil Nadu. The average family size ranged between greater than three members but less than four members was in Chhattisgarh, Delhi, Assam, Gujarat, Himachal Pradesh, Jharkhand, Manipur, Nagaland, West Bengal, Mizoram. Chandigarh was the only state where average family size ranged between greater than four members but less than five members.

Table 2.3.1: Average Family Size of Round 1, 2 and 3

(in Numbers)

State-wise Average Family Size of Round 1		
No. of States/UTs	***States/UTs***	***Average Family Size***
13	Bihar, Haryana, Karnataka, Kerala, Maharashtra, Meghalaya, Odisha, Punjab, Tripura, Uttar Pradesh, Uttrakhand, Goa, Tamil Nadu	>2 - <3
10	Chhattisgarh, Delhi, Assam, Gujarat, Himachal Pradesh, Jharkhand, Manipur, Nagaland, West Bengal, Mizoram	> 3 - < 4
1	Chandigarh	> 4 - < 5
State-wise Average Family Size of Round 2		
No. of States/UTs	***States/UTs***	***Average Family Size***
8	Delhi, Kerala, Maharashtra, Meghalaya, Odisha, Punjab, Uttar Pradesh, Uttrakhand	>2 - <3
9	Bihar, Chandigarh, Chhattisgarh, Gujarat, Haryana, Himachal Pradesh, Jharkhand, Nagaland, West Bengal	> 3 - < 4
State-wise Average Family Size of Round 3		
No. of States	***States***	***Average Family Size***
2	Haryana, Punjab	>2 - <3
3	Delhi, Kerala, Uttar Pradesh	> 3 - < 4

Source: Author's calculation.
Note: Average family size data obtained from www.rsby.gov.in.

In round 2, it was found that there were eight states having average family size greater than two members but less than three members viz. Delhi, Kerala, Maharashtra, Meghalaya, Odisha, Punjab, Uttar Pradesh, Uttrakhand and nine states had average family size between greater than three members but less than four members viz. Bihar, Chandigarh, Chhattisgarh, Gujarat, Haryana, Himachal Pradesh, Jharkhand, Nagaland, West Bengal. In round 2 and round 3 the average family size ranging between greater than four members but less than five members was not found in any state. In round 3, it was found that Haryana and Punjab had average family size which ranged between greater than two members but less than three members and three states viz. Delhi, Kerala and Uttar Pradesh had average family size greater than three members but less than four members. It was found that maximum number of average family size of RSBY beneficiaries was in range between greater than two members but less than three members and greater than three members but less than four members.

2.3.2 State-wise Average Claim, Conversion, Hospitalisation and Burnout Ratio

The state-wise average claim ratio, conversion ratio, hospitalisation ratio and burnout ratio have been depicted in Figure 2.3.3. The average claim ratio for round one was 62.12 per cent which increased to 110.55 per cent in round two due to proper implementation of RSBY to BPL population in various states. This proves that the BPL families availed themselves of the benefits and were satisfied with the services and benefits of the schemes as the claim ratio increased during the second year. It was 98.79 per cent in round three.

The average conversion ratio of round one was 54.1 per cent which increased to 56.67 per cent in round three. The increase in conversion ratio reveals that the outreach of the scheme to BPL population was positive and enrollment and utilisation of hospitalisation facilities raised the conversion over the years. The hospitalisation ratio in the first round was 1.81 per cent which proved that BPL families utilised the scheme and properly availed the hospitalisation benefits. The average hospitalisation ratio of round two was 2.64 per cent implying thereby that hospitalisation was more in these states as compared to the first year. The positive impact of RSBY was self-evident. Hospitalisation ratio went upto 6.05 per cent during the third round in the states, reflecting a quantum leap. The average expense ratio in round one was 72.84 per cent which means that the insurance companies enjoyed the profits during that period. The burnout ratio increased to 107.26 per cent in round two which showed losses to insurers in this round and more benefits for the beneficiaries.

(in Percentage)

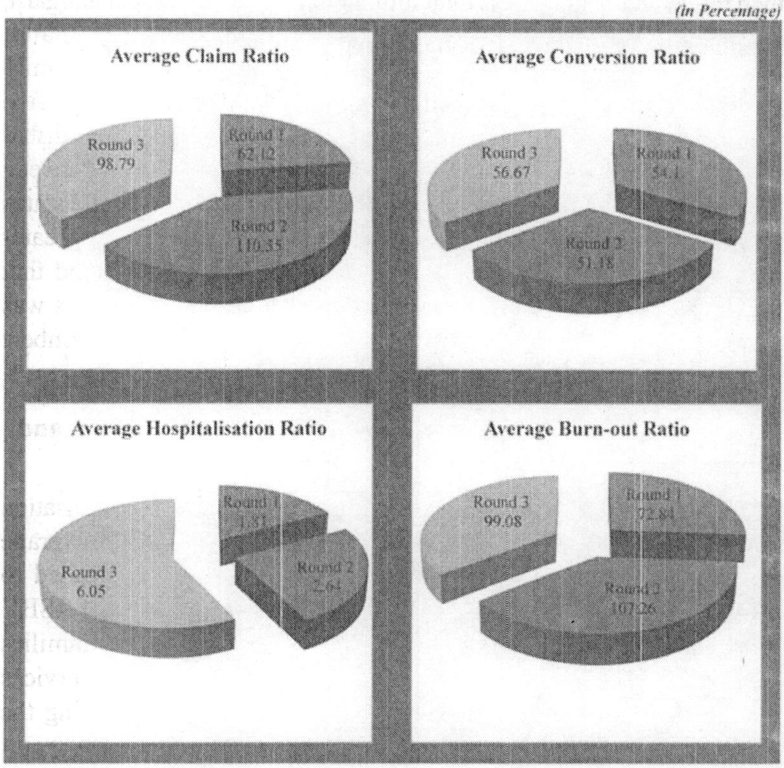

Source: Author's self-construction.

Note: Claim, Conversion, Hospitalisation and Burnout ratios computed from data obtained from Ministry of Health and Family Welfare.

Figure 2.3.3: State-wise Average Claim, Conversion, Hospitalisation and Burnout Ratio of Round 1, 2 and 3.

This increase in burn-out ratio is a function of decreasing premium and increasing hospitalisation. In round three, there was an average total expense ratio of 99.08 per cent implying that 0.02 per cent of the total premium remained with the insurer after expenses. Nominal profit was found in the third round. The burnout ratio of third round revealed that beneficiaries availed the hospitalisation services happily and felt satisfied with the scheme.

2.3.3 State-wise Comparison of Claim Ratio

Table 2.3.2 deals with the comparison of claim ratio of round one, two and three. In round 1, 12 states had less than 50 per cent claim ratio viz. Assam, Chhattisgarh, Goa, Jharkhand, Karnataka, Maharashtra, Chandigarh, Meghalaya, Odisha, Punjab, Tamil Nadu, Uttrakhand.

Table 2.3.2: State-wise Comparison of Claim Ratio of Round 1, 2 and 3

Percentage of State-wise Claim Ratio - Round 1		
No. of States/UTs	*States/ UTs*	*Percentage*
12	Assam, Chhattisgarh, Goa, Jharkhand, Karnataka, Maharashtra, Chandigarh, Meghalaya, Odisha, Punjab, Tamil Nadu, Uttrakhand	<50
9	Bihar, Gujarat, Haryana, West Bengal, Himachal Pradesh Kerala, Mizoram, Tripura, Uttar Pradesh	51-100
2	Delhi, Nagaland	101-150
1	Manipur	151-200
Percentage of State-wise Claim Ratio - Round 2		
No. of States/UTs	*States/ UTs*	*Percentage*
11	Chhattisgarh, Delhi, Gujarat, Jharkhand, Meghalaya, Chandigarh, Nagaland, Odisha, Punjab, Uttar Pradesh, West Bengal	51-100
3	Bihar, Haryana, Maharashtra	101-150
2	Kerala, Uttrakhand	151-200
1	Himachal Pradesh	251-300
Percentage of State-wise Claim Ratio - Round 3		
No. of States	*States*	*Percentage*
1	Punjab	<50
3	Delhi, Haryana, Kerala	51-100
1	Uttar Pradesh	101-150

Source: Author's calculation.

*Note:*Claim ratios computed from data obtained from Ministry of Health and Family Welfare.

The claims ratio ranged between 51-100 per cent in nine states viz. Bihar, Gujarat, Haryana, West Bengal, Himachal Pradesh, Kerala, Mizoram, Tripura, Uttar Pradesh. Delhi and Nagaland had claim ratio in the range of 101-150 per cent and the claim ratio ranged between 151-200 per cent was only in Manipur. The claim ratio ranging between 201-250 per cent and 251-300 per cent was not in any state.

Chhattisgarh, Delhi, Gujarat, Jharkhand, Meghalaya, Chandigarh, Nagaland, Odisha, Punjab, Uttar Pradesh, West Bengal and claim ratios of three states viz. Bihar, Haryana and Maharashtra were in the range of 101-150 per cent. Kerala and Uttrakhand were in the range of 151-200 per cent and Himachal Pradesh was the only state in the range of 250-300 per cent. There was not even a single state in the range between 201-250. In round two, the maximum claim was of Himachal Pradesh in the range of 250-300 per cent whereas, the claim ratio of Himachal Pradesh in round one was in the range of 50-100 per cent which indicated that there was a good response from BPL population for enrollment and utilisation of services of RSBY. This further proved that the BPL families were satisfied with the services and benefits of the schemes. In round three, the highest claim ratio in the range of 101-150 per cent was in Uttar Pradesh and Punjab had the claim ratio of less than 50 per cent. Delhi, Haryana and Kerala had claim ratio in the range of 51-100 per cent. The claim ratio ranging between 151-200 per cent, 201-250 per cent and 251-300 per cent was not in any state. From the comparison of claim ratio of three rounds, it was found that that the second round was more beneficial to BPL families and large number of BPL families utilised the benefits of the scheme.

2.3.4 State-wise Comparison of Conversion Ratio

Table 2.3.3 shows the comparison of conversion ratio of round 1, 2 and 3. In round 1, less than 20 per cent conversion ratio was observed in Assam and Delhi. The conversion ratio of Mizoram, Punjab and

Table 2.3.3: State-wise Comparison of Conversion Ratio of Round 1, 2 and 3

State-wise Conversion Ratio - Round 1		
No. of States/UTs	*States/ UTs*	*Percentage*
2	Assam, Delhi	<20
3	Mizoram, Punjab, Tamil Nadu	21-40
12	Bihar, Chhattisgarh, Goa, Haryana, Jharkhand, Karnataka, Kerala, Maharashtra, Meghalaya, Odisha, Uttar Pradesh, Uttrakhand	41-60
5	Gujarat, Manipur, Nagaland, West Bengal, Chandigarh	61-80
2	Himachal Pradesh, Tripura	81-100

(Contd...)

State-wise Conversion Ratio - Round 2		
No. of States/UTs	***States/ UTs***	***Percentage***
1	Uttar Pradesh	21-40
10	Bihar, Delhi, Haryana, Jharkhand, Maharashtra, Meghalaya, Odisha, Punjab, Uttrakhand, Chandigarh	41-60
6	Chhattisgarh, Gujarat, Himachal Pradesh, Kerala, Nagaland, West Bengal	61-80
State-wise Conversion Ratio - Round 3		
No. of States	***States***	***Percentage***
1	Delhi	<20
1	Uttar Pradesh	21-40
2	Punjab, Haryana	41-60
1	Kerala	61-80

Source: Author's calculation.

Note: Conversion ratio computed from data obtained from Ministry of Health and Family Welfare.

Tamil Nadu were in the range of 21-40 per cent. The conversion ratio ranging between 41-60 per cent was in 12 states viz. Bihar, Chhattisgarh, Goa, Haryana, Jharkhand, Karnataka, Kerala, Maharashtra, Meghalaya, Odisha, Uttar Pradesh and Uttrakhand. Five states viz. Gujarat, Manipur, Nagaland, West Bengal and Chandigarh showed the conversion ratio in the range of 61-80 per cent. The maximum outreach of scheme was shown by Himachal Pradesh and Tripura in the range of 81-100 per cent.

In round 2, the conversion ratio ranged between 21-80 per cent in 17 states. The significant variations were witnessed across states. The conversion ratio of Uttar Pradesh was in the range of 21-40. Bihar, Delhi, Haryana, Jharkhand, Maharashtra, Meghalaya, Odisha, Punjab, Uttrakhand and Chandigarh showed the conversion ratio between 41-60 per cent. The conversion ratios of less than 20 per cent and 81-100 per cent were not in any state. The conversion ratio of six states viz. Chhattisgarh, Gujarat, Himachal Pradesh, Kerala, Nagaland and West Bengal were in the range of 61-80 per cent. In the second round, the conversion ratio of RSBY was good in various states which showed the positive impact of the scheme. In round 3, Delhi was the only state which had shown less than 20 per cent conversion. The conversion of

Uttar Pradesh was in the range of 21-40 per cent whereas Punjab and Haryana showed the conversion ratio in the range of 41-60 per cent. Kerala was the only state which had maximum outreach of the scheme in round three ranging between 61-80 per cent.The increase in conversion ratio revealed that the impact of RSBY on poor people was significant while registration and utilisation was indoor treatment facilities had increased the conversion over the years.

2.3.5 State-wise Comparison of Hospitalisation Ratio

Table 2.3.4 explains the comparison of hospitalisation ratio of first, second and third rounds. In round one, 15 states viz. Assam, Chattisgarh, Goa, Jharkhand, Karnataka, Chandigarh, Meghalaya, Punjab, West Bengal, Uttrakhand, Bihar, Himachal Pradesh, Mizoram, Maharashtra showed the hospitalisation ratio of less than two per cent. The hospitalisation ratio of eight states viz. Gujarat, Haryana, Manipur, Nagaland, Tamil Nadu, Tripura, Delhi and Uttar Pradesh was in the range of greater than two per cent but less than four per cent. Kerala was the only state which showed the hospitalisation ratio in the range of greater than four per cent but less than six per cent. The hospitalisation ratio ranging between greater than six per cent but less than eight per cent was not in any state. The hospitalisation ratio in the first round proved that poor people received the benefits of the scheme to a great extent. Registration of beneficiaries when increased during the very first year hospitalisation ratio was used to find the proportion of beneficiaries vis-à-vis the enrollment figures. This tool can be based reliably on evaluate the scheme.

In round two, nine states viz. Nagaland, Chandigarh, Bihar, Chhattisgarh, Gujarat, Jharkhand, Meghalaya, Odisha and West Bengal showed the hospitalisation ratio of less than two per cent. The hospitalisation ratio of Haryana, Maharashtra, Punjab, Uttar Pradesh, Uttrakhand and Himachal Pradesh was in the range of greater than two per cent but less than four per cent. The hospitalisation ratio of Delhi was in the range of greater than four per cent but less than six per cent and Kerala was the only state which showed the highest hospitalisation ratio in round two ranging between greater than six per cent but less than eight per cent.

Table 2.3.4: State-wise Comparison of Hospitalisation Ratio of Round 1, 2 and 3

State-wise Hospitalisation Ratio - Round 1		
No. of States/UTs	***States/ UTs***	***Percentage***
15	Assam, Chhattisgarh, Goa, Jharkhand, Karnataka, Chandigarh, Meghalaya, Odisha, Punjab, West Bengal, Uttrakhand, Bihar, Himachal Pradesh, Mizoram, Maharashtra	<2
8	Gujarat, Haryana, Manipur, Nagaland, Tamil Nadu, Tripura, Delhi, Uttar Pradesh	>2 - <4
1	Kerala	>4 - <6
State-wise Hospitalisation Ratio - Round 2		
No. of States/UTs	***States/ UTs***	***Percentage***
9	Nagaland, Chandigarh, Bihar, Chhattisgarh, Gujarat, Jharkhand, Meghalaya, Odisha, West Bengal	<2
6	Haryana, Maharashtra, Punjab, Uttar Pradesh, Uttrakhand, Himachal Pradesh	>2 - <4
1	Delhi	>4 - <6
1	Kerala	>6 - <8
State-wise Hospitalisation Ratio - Round 3		
No. of States	***States***	***Percentage***
1	Punjab	<2
3	Delhi, Haryana, Uttar Pradesh	>2 - <4
1	Kerala	>6 - <8

Source: Author's calculation.

Note: Hospitalisation ratio computed from data obtained from Ministry of Health and Family Welfare.

In the third round, Punjab showed the hospitalisation ratio of less than two per cent. The hospitalisation ratio of Delhi, Haryana and Uttar Pradesh was in the range of greater than two per cent but less than four per cent and Kerala was the only state which showed the ratio between greater than six per cent but less than eight per cent. The hospitalisation ratio ranging between greater than four per cent but less than 6 per cent was not in any state. The average hospitalisation ratio of round two implied that hospitalisation ratio was more as compared to the first year. The positive impact of RSBY was self-evident. Hospitalisation ratio went upto greater than six per cent but less than eight per cent during the second and third rounds in the states. Evidently the indoor treatment rate has been improving with the passage of time which proves that the scheme has influenced the lives of the poor people to a great extent in terms of healthcare and clearly demonstrated improvement in access to hospitalisation.

2.3.6 State-wise Comparison of Burn-out/Expense Ratio

Table 2.3.5 shows the comparison of burnout ratio of first, second and third rounds. The burnout ratio of Assam, Chhattisgarh, Goa, Odisha, Tamil Nadu, Uttrakhand, Chandigarh was less than 50 per cent whereas both the beneficiaries and the insurers were benefited. Fourteen states viz. Bihar, Gujarat, Haryana, West Bengal, Himachal Pradesh, Kerala, Mizoram, Tripura, Uttar Pradesh, Jharkhand, Karnataka, Maharashtra, Meghayala and Punjab had shown the burnout ratio ranging between 51-100 per cent.

Table 2.3.5: State-wise Comparison of Burnout Ratio of Round 1, 2 and 3

Percentage of State-wise Burnout Ratio - Round 1		
No. of States/UTs	*States/UTs*	*Percentage*
7	Assam, Chhattisgarh, Goa, Odisha, Tamil Nadu, Uttrakhand, Chandigarh	< 50
14	Bihar, Gujarat, Haryana, West Bengal, Himachal Pradesh, Kerala, Mizoram, Tripura, Uttar Pradesh, Jharkhand, Karnataka, Maharashtra, Meghayala, Punjab	51-100
2	Delhi, Nagaland	101-150
1	Manipur	151-200
Percentage of State-wise Burnout Ratio - Round 2		
No. of States/UTs	*States/UTs*	*Percentage*
11	Chhattisgarh, Delhi, Gujarat, Jharkhand, Meghalaya, Chandigarh, Nagaland, Odisha, Punjab, Uttar Pradesh, West Bengal	51-100
3	Bihar, Haryana, Maharashtra	101-150
3	Kerala, Uttrakhand, Himachal Pradesh	151-200

(Contd...)

Percentage of State-wise Burnout Ratio - Round 3		
No. of States	*States*	*Percentage*
4	Delhi, Haryana, Kerala, Punjab	51-100
1	Uttar Pradesh	101-150

Source: Author's calculation.

Note: Burnout ratio computed from data obtained from Ministry of Health and Family Welfare.

The burnout ratio of Delhi and Nagaland was in the range of 101-150 per cent whereas Manipur was the only state where it ranged between 151-200 per cent.

In round two, the burnout ratio ranged between 51-200 per cent and burnout ratio of less than 50 per cent was not in any state. The burnout ratio of 11 states viz. Chhattisgarh, Delhi, Gujarat, Jharkhand, Meghalaya, Chandigarh, Nagaland, Odisha, Punjab, Uttar Pradesh, West Bengal was in the range of 51-100. The burnout ratio of Bihar, Haryana, Maharashtra ranged between 101-150 per cent whereas, that of Kerala, Uttrakhand and Himachal Pradesh ranged between 151-200 per cent. In the very first year there was an affirmative response the claimants regarding the benefits of the scheme to the poor people. The increased of hospitalisation ratio because more and more people realise the value of joining the scheme. In round three, Delhi, Haryana, Kerala and Punjab had shown the burnout ratio ranging between 51-100 per cent whereas Uttar Pradesh was the only state with range of 101-150 per cent burnout ratio. The burnout ratios less than 50 per cent and 151-200 per cent were not in any state. The burnout ratio in respect of third phase revealed that poor people had availed medical care services with satisfaction and they were happy with the scheme. Different rounds showed that this ratio was increasing gradually.

2.3.7 RSBY Through Gender Lens

Due to biological differences males and females encounter different health hazards. Our social norms and expectations from people add to the problem. It is fact that females generally live longer than men. Lack of resources difference in capabilities, denial of rights deprived females from healthcare. One cannot speak of health insurance for them in a traditional world. If females are provided standard health- care this can ensure them justice and equality which they need the most.

Figure 2.3.4 reveals the gender-wise enrollment rate of round one, two and three. It is encouragingly to note that more and more women have offered themselves for registration. With the result, enrollment of women as a percentage of total increased from 39.7 per cent in round one to 48.1 per cent in round three. This shows that women were more enthusiastic about joining the RSBY. Availing of scheme also highlights the fact that women were reaping the benefits from this scheme. May be this was due to the hidden demand for healthcare in the society.

(in Percentage)

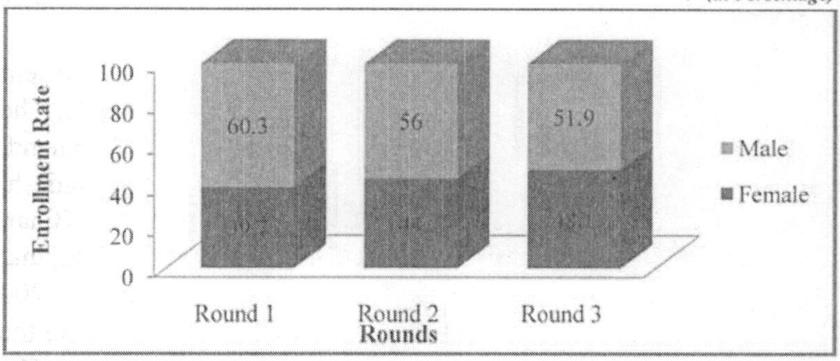

Source: Author's self-construction.
Note: Gender-wise enrollment data obtained from www.rsby.gov.in.

Figure 2.3.4: Gender-wise Enrollment Rate of Round 1, 2 and 3.

Gender-based data regarding use of indoor treatment is very surprising. Since this scheme covers child birth in its preview, the females are increasing attracted towards the scheme. It comes into light that indoor treatment ratio for women were 39.70 per cent while it was 60.30 per cent for men in the first round of the scheme. The third round saw 48.10 per cent of women and 51.90 per cent of men as beneficiaries. In absolute terms the number of women was low but when they are enrolled they used the services more often than men. The fact is encouraging because it points that the scheme is serving the people for whom it was meant.

SECTION IV

2.4 Insurer-wise Impact of RSBY on BPL Population in India

This section focuses on four key performance indicators (KPIs) – Claims Ratio (utility to the beneficiaries), Conversion Ratio (to measure depth of outreach), Hospitalisation Ratio (to gauge utilisation) and

Total Expense Ratio (to evaluate profitability to the insurer). These KPIs have been analysed from aggregated insurer-wise data for the first and second years of operations for ten general insurers and for the third year for four insurers. Primarily the success of health insurance schemes are very much dependent on the co-operation rendered by the insurers because they were the major stakeholders in the whole exercise. Ten general insurance companies were actively involved in implementation of RSBY that completed the first round (2008-09) of operations with great success and raised hopes of the stakeholders in this venture, including the policy-makers and the beneficiaries. The same general insurers extended whole hearted co-operation in the second round also (2009-10) and four of them joined hands with RSBY planners to execute it in the third round (2010-11). This reflects the comfort level of the insurance companies and their belief in the long-term commitment of the government in respect of RSBY scheme.

2.4.1 Insurer-wise Number of States

Figure 2.4.1 shows number of states per insurer in three rounds. The distribution of general insurance companies of round one was in

(in Numbers)

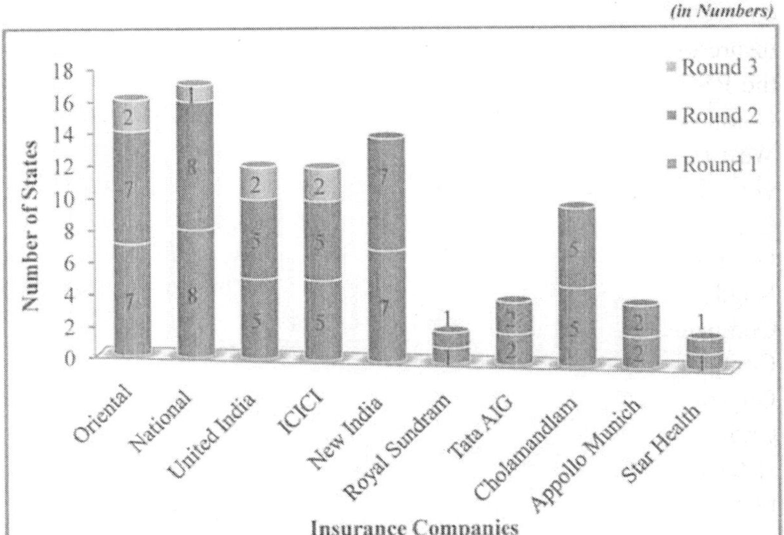

Source: Author's self-construction.

Note: Insurer-wise number of states data obtained from Ministry of Health and Family Welfare.

Figure 2.4.1: Number of States per Insurer of Round 1, 2 and 3.

24 states, round two in 17 states and round three in five states. There were four public and six private general insurance players participated in the implementation of RSBY scheme in round 1.

National Insurance Company (a public general insurer) was involved in eight states viz. Assam, Karnataka, Maharashtra, Mizoram, Punjab, West Bengal, Tripura and Chandigarh. Oriental Insurance Company was actively involved in seven states viz. Bihar, Chhattisgarh, Delhi, Gujarat, Jharkhand, Maharashtra, Punjab and United India Insurance participated in five states viz. Bihar, Kerala, Tamil Nadu, West Bengal and Uttrakhand. New India Assurance Company was actively involved in seven states viz. Goa, Gujarat, Himachal Pradesh, Maharashtra, Manipur, Nagaland and Odisha,whereas, the private health insurer, ICICI Lombard General Insurance Company covered five states viz. Bihar, Gujarat, Haryana, Maharashtra and Uttar Pradesh and Cholamandlam General Insurance Company also covered five states viz. Bihar, Gujarat, Jharkhand, Maharashtra and West Bengal and only Uttrakhand was covered by Star Health and Allied Insurance Company. Royal Sundram Alliance Insurance Company provided services to Bihar only and Tata AIG General Insurance Company covered Chhattisgarh and Maharashtra, whereas Meghalaya and Nagaland were two states covered by Apollo Munich Health Insurance Company. Ten general insurers (four public and six private) moved hand in hand to implement the RSBY scheme in 17 states in second round. National Insurance Company showed its presence in three states viz. Bihar, Haryana and West Bengal. Oriental Insurance Company also covered three states viz. Chhattisgarh, Delhi and Uttar Pradesh. United India Insurance Company covered four states viz. Punjab, Kerala, Uttar Pradesh and Uttrakhand. New India Insurance was active in Himachal Pradesh, Nagaland and West Bengal. Royal Sundram Alliance Insurance Company covered only Bihar and ICICI Lombard General Insurance Company actively participated in seven states viz. Punjab, Haryana, Gujarat, Maharashtra, Odisha, Uttar Pradesh and Chandigarh. Cholamandlam MS General Insurance Company took care of three states viz. Gujarat, Jharkhand and Maharashtra. The only state Haryana, two states viz. Maharashtra and Meghalaya and one state Maharashtra were covered by Star Health and Allied Insurance Company, Apollo Munich Health Insurance Company and Tata AIG General Insurance Company respectively. There were three public and only one private general insurer dealing with health insurance in five states under RSBY in round three. Oriental Insurance Company covered Delhi and Uttar Pradesh, United India Insurance Company covered Uttar Pradesh and Kerala whereas, National Insurance Company covered only Haryana. ICICI Lombard General Insurance Company participated in Punjab and Uttar Pradesh.

The total premium paid to the insurance companies by central and state governments was ₹ 1271 crore in the first round. ICICI Lombard General Insurance Company, (private general insurer) received ₹ 495 crore followed by Oriental Insurance Company (public general insurer) of ₹ 169.47 crore and the least premium ₹ 45 crore was of Star Health and Allied Insurance Company. ₹ 633 crore were collected as premium in round two. Once again ICICI Lombard General Insurance Company claimed a lion's share of ₹ 148.67 crore followed by ₹ 133.94 crore of United India insurance Company in the round two. The least premium collection (₹ 3.67 crore) was of Tata AIG. In round three, total premium revenue of four insurers was to the tune of ₹ 295 crore. Since only five states had completed the round three so the number of BPL families served fell dramatically as was revealed by decrease in premium. ICICI Lombard General Insurance Company was the leading company in round one and two and United India Insurance Company in round three.

2.4.2 Insurer-wise Comparison of Claim Ratio of Round 1, 2 and 3

The insurer-wise comparison of claims ratio of round 1, 2 and 3 is shown in Figure 2.4.2. The claim ratio of round one was 63.78 per cent which increased to 110.55 per cent in round 2. However, it was 100.21 per cent in round 3. The utilisation of RSBY scheme increased during the years with a positive impact on the beneficiaries.

In round one, United India Insurance Company, a public general insurer and ICICI Lombard General Insurance Company, a private general insurer had highest claim ratio. The lowest claim ratio was shown by Tata AIG (27.44 per cent) followed by Star Health and Allied Insurance Company (29.36 per cent). In round two, United India Insurance Company had highest claim ratio of 153.36 per cent followed by National Insurance Company (139.11 per cent). New India Assurance Company showed least claim ratio among the public general insurers. Tata AIG General Insurance Company, a private general

(in Percentage)

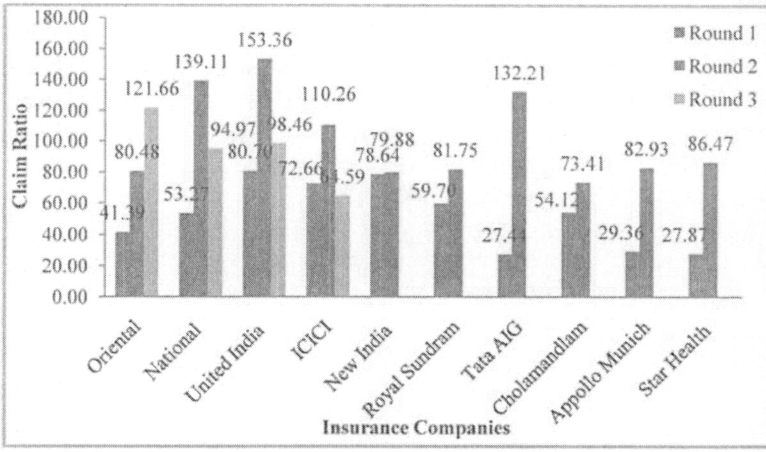

Source: Author's self-construction.

Note: Insurer-wise claim ratio computed from data obtained from Ministry of Health and Family Welfare.

Figure 2.4.2: Insurer-wise Comparison of Claim Ratio of Round 1, 2 and 3.

insurer recorded 132.21 per cent claim ratio followed by 110.26 per cent of ICICI Lombard General Insurance Company. The increase in claim ratio resulted into increase in take up ratio among beneficairies which further showed the positive impact of RSBY on BPL population. In round three, Oriental Insurance showed claim ratio of 121.66 per cent and ICICI Lombard General Insurance Company showed claim ratio 64.59 per cent. Two insurers had claim ratio in the range of 95-100 per cent and ICICI Lombard General Insurance Company had claim ratio of more than 60 per cent which revealed the proper utilisation of RSBY among beneficiaries.

2.4.3 Insurer-wise Comparison of Conversion Ratio of Round 1, 2 and 3

Figure 2.4.3 shows the comparison of conversion ratio of general insurers during rounds one, two and three. The conversion ratio decreased marginally from 54.10 per cent in round two to 51.18 per cent in round two and slightly increased to 56.67 per cent in round three.

In round one, there were huge differences across public and private general insurers. Cholamandlam MS General Insurance Company had the highest conversion ratio of 243.30 per cent and the least conversion ratio of 3.80 per cent was of Tata AIG. The conversion ratio of six general insurers ranged between 50-70 per cent and two insurers had more than 100 per cent conversion ratio which proves the possible impact on the lives of the poor people. In second round, New India Insurance showed highest conversion ratio of 68.07 per cent and the least conversion ratio of 34.89 per cent was shown by Star Health and Allied Insurance Company. Oriental Insurance Company, National Insurance Company, Royal Sundram Alliance Insurance Company, Cholamandlam MS General Insurance Company and Apollo Munich Health Insurance Company had conversion ratio in the range of 50-60 per cent.

(in Percentage)

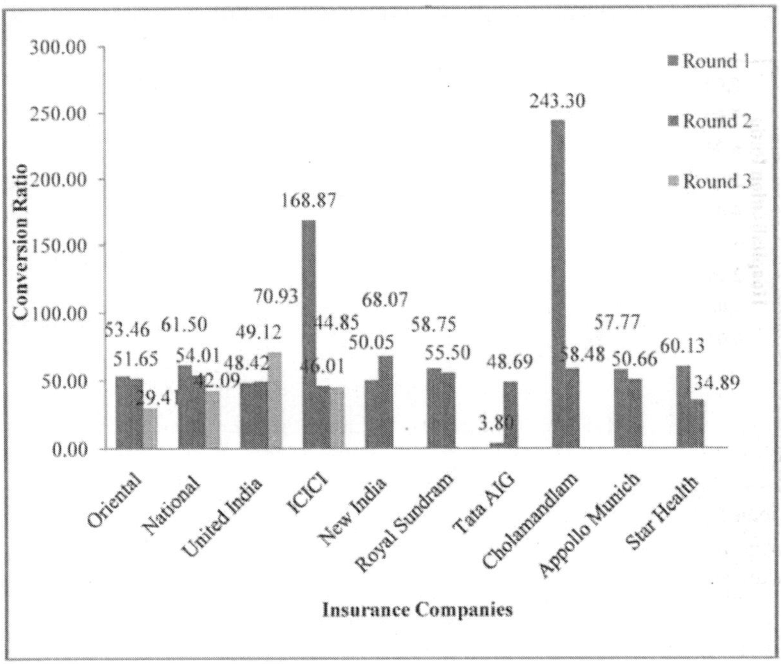

Source: Author's self-construction.

Note: Insurer-wise conversion ratio computed from data obtained from Ministry of Health and Family Welfare.

Figure 2.4.3: Insurer-wise Comparison of Conversion Ratio of Round 1, 2 and 3.

There were significant variations across general insurers. The highest conversion ratio of 70.93 was of United India Insurance Company and the least conversion ratio of 29.41 per cent was of Oriental Insurance Company. The number of poor families enrolling under the scheme grew day by day and sizeable number of them went in for indoor medical treatment due to which the conversion ratio showed an upward trend.

2.4.4 Insurer-wise Comparison of Hospitalisation Ratio of Round 1, 2 and 3

The comparison of hospitalisation ratio of three rounds has been shown in Figure 2.4.4. United India Insurance Company was the leading company in three years with highest hospitalisation ratio. This makes it the best performer during the three years.

(in Percentage)

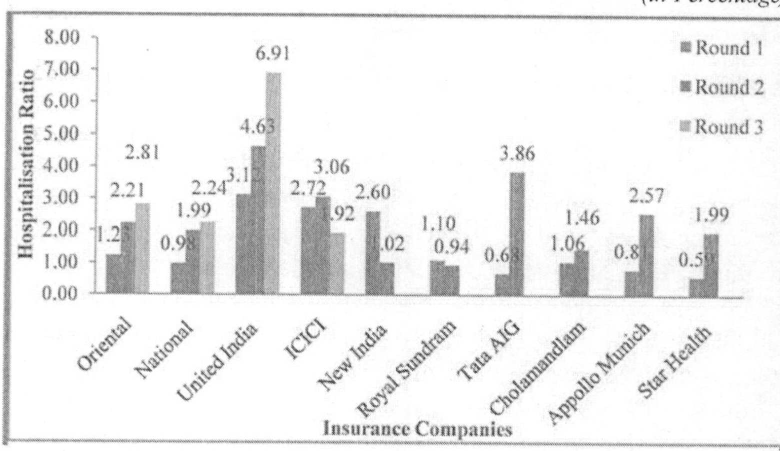

Source: Author's self-construction.

Note: Hospitalisation ratio computed from data obtained from Ministry of Health and Family Welfare.

Figure 2.4.4: Insurer-wise Comparison of Hospitalisation Ratio of Round 1, 2 and 3.

ICICI Lombard General Insurance Company, a private general insurer showed highest hospitalisation ratio in round one and two but decreased in round three due to tough competition. With the passage of time hospitalisation ratio got a fillip in all the three rounds. The efforts of administration regarding spreading of awareness in rural people and in villages bore fruit and they felt attracted towards the scheme. Taking up individually, except New India Insurance Company and Royal Sundram Alliance Insurance Company where hospitalisation ratio fell, in case of all other general insurance companies, there was a hike. The highest increase was of Tata AIG General Insurance Company (from 0.68 per cent during the first year to 3.86 per cent in the second round). Star Health and Allied Insurance Company, which was failed in case of hospitalisation at less than 0.59 per cent, grew to 1.99 per cent during the second round. The hospitalisation ratio had increased unexpectedly during the second year. As against an average of 1.84 per cent during the first year, it reached 2.64 per cent and 5.87 per cent in second and third rounds respectively. The comparison of hospitalisation ratios during the second and third round shows that awareness level, use of scheme and penetration thereof improved considerably which is a proof of positive influence of scheme on poor people.

2.4.5 Insurer-wise Comparison of Burnout Ratio of Round 1, 2 and 3

Burnout ratio means the expenditure by insurers taken as percentage of expenditure done on paying hospitals for paying claims, procuring smart card and service tax against money received as premium. EIC activities led to overwhelming response from public which result into more and more hospitalisation. Consequently, burnout ratio crossed the average of first round which was 73.6 per cent and reached to 107.26 per cent in the second round and 100.6 per cent in third round. Only a few states succeeded in completely the third round. Data pertaining to them is not sufficient enough to reach wide conclusion. There was much for all the stakeholders to learn from their experiences. The processes and systems initiated during the scheme have taken roots and the expansion of the scheme has present new issues and problems that deserve utmost attention. As compared to the last two rounds, the first round paid the insurance company a rich dividend. In the other rounds it was the beneficiaries who got better services while the insurance companies were not big gainers.

Figure 2.4.5 compares the burnout ratio of three rounds. In round one, United India Insurance, a public general insurer showed the highest burnout ratio (86.58 per cent) followed by New India Insurance Company (84.57 per cent). Among the private general insurers ICICI Lombard General Insurance Company showed the maximum burnout ratio (80.10 per cent) followed by Cholamandlam MS General insurance Company (67.26 per cent).The health insurance services were availed by the masses to great level. The least ratio of 47.89 per cent was shown by Tata AIG General Insurance Company.

In round two, the highest ratio was shown by United India Insurance Company (136.26 per cent) followed by National Insurance Company (126.35 per cent). Tata AIG General Insurance Company, a private insurer showed highest burnout ratio more than 100 per cent.

(in Percentage)

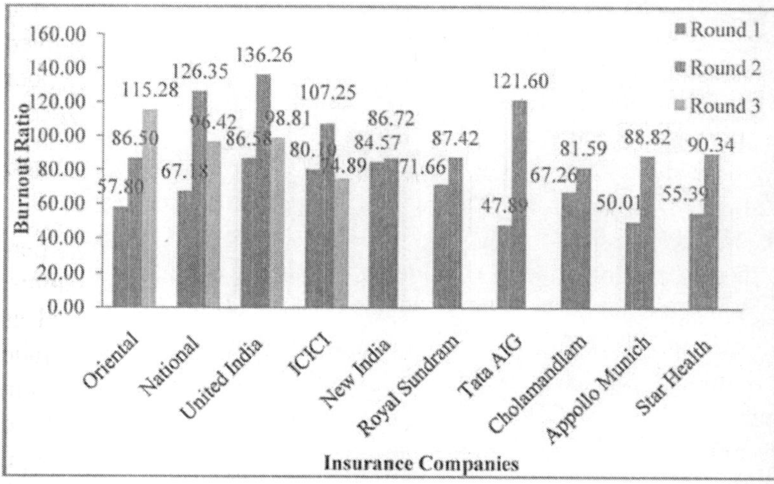

Source: Author's self-construction.

Note: Insurer-wise burnout ratio computed from data obtained from Ministry of Health and Family Welfare.

Figure 2.4.5: Insurer-wise Comparison of Burnout Ratio of Round 1, 2 and 3.

There was an increase in the burnout ratio in respect of all insurance companies in the first, second and third rounds. May be the poor people found the scheme very attractive and beneficial and were benefited under the scheme to a great extent. In round three, Oriental Insurance Company led with 115.28 per cent followed by United India Insurance Company (98.81 per cent). There were only four companies that showed average burnout ratio of more than 100 per cent. The trend was detrimental to the interest of insurance companies but very congenial for the welfare of the poor people.

SECTION V

2.5 Conclusion

As a result majority of Indians have to bear the cost of medical treatment for their own pockets. It is evident from National Health Accounts data that only 20 per cent of health expenditure is borne by government while almost the entire amount is paid by the individuals from their own pockets. Nowhere in the world is visible is such a situation. Government of India health spending has to be estimated to about 4.5 per cent of GDP while expenditure on healthcare is meagre 0.9 per cent of GDP. Lack of funds, faulty infrastructure, low quality healthcare and poor accessibility to the rural people characterise public healthcare system. The Government of India (GOI) has already made provisions of hospital insurance by subsidiary premium for the poor population. Therefore, in 2008, the Government of India introduced the "Rashtriya Swasthya Bima Yojna" (RSBY). RSBY is uniquely mandated to cover the entire BPL population irrespective of occupational distribution and helps to reduce out-of-pocket expenditure on healthcare and lessen a considerable financial burden on the poor. It has been an important step to supplement the efforts being made to provide quality healthcare to the poor and under-privileged population. It covers hospitalisation costs up to ₹ 30,000 per annum per household and scheme is jointly funded by the central and state governments in the ratio of 75:25 per cent with a small contribution from the beneficiary household.

Healthcare in India is financed through individual out-of-pocket payments, central and state government tax revenues, external aid and other sources. National health accounts data reveal that the government sector (central, state and local) account for only 20 per cent of total health expenditures, external aid via the voluntary sector account for two per cent and 78 per cent take the form of out-of-pocket payments – one of the highest percentages in the world. To reduce out-of-pocket expenditure on healthcare and lessen a considerable financial burden on the poor, a national health insurance scheme, Rashtriya Swasthya Bima Yojna (RSBY) launched by Ministry of Labour and Employment in 2007 has been an important step to supplement the efforts being made to provide quality healthcare to the poor and under-privileged population.

RSBY is a central level health insurance scheme for BPL families with easy access and covering the financial risk. The coverage of the scheme is up to ₹ 30,000 per year per household. A beneficiary and his family combined has to pay the registration fee of ₹ 30 on yearly basis and premium responsibility is of 750 is borne by the Central and State Governments in the ratio of 3:1. The scheme is jointly funded by the central and the state governments. In January 2014, total 30 states/UTs enrolled with RSBY and the total BPL families were 77.80 millions, out of which 40.13 million families (51.6 per cent) enrolled by using smart cards. The total districts in thirty states/UTs were 645 and 536 districts enrolled for RSBY scheme out of which in 468 districts have completed their enrollment and 38 districts were in progress with RSBY Scheme. About 40.13 million smart cards (covering 140.45 million persons) were distributed to the beneficiaries. The total healthcare providers in RSBY were 11,565 out of which 7,328 were private and 4,237 were public hospitals. The maximum hospitals were in Uttar Pradesh i.e., 1,984 out of which 63.2 per cent were private hospitals and 36.8 per cent were public.

Efforts have been made to examine the state-wise impact of Rashtriya Swasthya Bima Yojna on below poverty line population through claim ratio, conversion ratio, hospitalisation ratio and burnout ratio. The districts in which scheme started its implementation in 2008, the average premium decreased from ₹ 607 during round one to ₹ 518 in round three, in year 2009 from ₹ 600 in round one to ₹ 513 in round three, in year 2010 from ₹ 533 to ₹ 412 in round three.

The study focused on four key performance indicators (KPIs) – Claims Ratio (utilisation by beneficiaries), Conversion Ratio (a tool for measuring outreach), Hospitalisation Ratio (an indicator of utilisation of healthcare) and Total Expense Ratio (a parameter to judge profit to the insurance company). These KPIs were analysed from state-wise data for the first year of operations for 24 states, in the second year for 17 states and in the third year for five states. In round one, the statewise claim ratio of 24 states was 62.12 per cent which goes to 110.55 per cent in round two and it was 98.79 per cent in round three.

The average conversion ratio of round one was 54.1 per cent which increased to 56.67 per cent in round three. The average expense ratio in round one was 72.84 per cent which increased to 107.26 per cent in round two and third year witnessed a drop in average expense ratio to 99.08 per cent.The state-wise comparison of claim ratio explained that in round one, 12 states had less than 50 per cent claim ratio and 51-100 per cent, 101-150 per cent and 151-200 per cent claim ratio were in nine, two and one state respectively. In round two, the claim ratio ranging between 51-100 per cent, 101-150 per cent, 151-200 per cent, 250-300 per cent was in nine, three, two and one state respectively. In round three, claim ratio of 101-150 per cent and 51-100 per cent both was only in two states where, as, only one state had claim ratio of less than 50 per cent.

From the comparison of hospitalisation ratio of three rounds, it has been found that in round one, 15, 8 and 1 state have shown the hospitalisation ratio of less than two per cent, greater than two per cent but less than four per cent, greater than four per cent but less than six per cent. In round two, the hospitalisation ratio of less than two per cent, greater than two per cent but less than four per cent, greater than four per cent but less than six per cent and greater than six per cent but less than eight per cent have shown in nine, six, one and one state respectively. In third round one, three and one state has shown the hospitalisation ratio of less than two per cent, greater than two per cent but less than four per cent and greater than six per cent but less than eight per cent. An analysis of burnout ratio shows that in round one, the burnout ratio of 7, 14, 2 and 1 state was less than 50 per cent, 51-100 per cent, 101-150 per cent and 151-200 per cent respectively. In round two, the burnout ratio of 11, 3 and 3 states ranged between 51-100 per cent 101-150 per cent and 151-200 per cent. In round three, burnout ratio ranged between 51-100 per cent and 101-150 per cent showed in four and one state. The burnout ratio of third round revealed that the beneficiaries had availed the hospitalisation services happily and were satisfied with the scheme.

RSBY has been a landmark development in the direction of provision of quality healthcare to the poor and giving a business to all key stakeholder i.e. insurance companies, hospitals, smart card service provides and TPAs. The impact of RSBY on the lives of the BPL families revealed that most of beneficiaries felt satisfied by the benefits accrued to them under the scheme and hospitalisation rate increased over time showing a positive impact of the scheme. The RSBY scheme is a guidance and supportive factor for rendering free hospitalisation facilities to the BPL population in India and also followed by other countries. Therefore, it comes into light that RSBY is giving a positive impact, as more and more BPL population registered and availing the benefits from the scheme over the time.

Chapter - 3

Rashtriya Swasthya Bima Yojna and Other Public Sector Health Insurance Schemes

Before the advent of government sponsored health insurance schemes (GSHISs), almost all public expenditure was meant for public delivery system. Since there was low public health financing, significant responsibility issues in the system and sizeable from the pocket expenditure by the poor patients. GSHISs came as an alternative of utilising and distribution of funds for the purpose. GSHISs have initiated a sort of new activities for administration, utilisation and management of public health resources. These changes serve as a new foundation for Indian public health delivery system. To focus on the coming issues in this sector, four GSHISs were reviewed so that the results obtained may be serving as guidance to all the stakeholders and policymakers. The objective of this chapter is to compare Rasthriya Swasthya Bima Yojna (RSBY) (central one) with other public sector health Insurance schemes viz. Rajiv Aarogyasri scheme (RAS) of Andhra Pradesh, Vajpayee Arogyasri scheme (VAS) of Karnataka and Chief Minister Kalaignar Health Insurance scheme (CMKHIS) of Tamil Nadu. The chapter has been divided into four sections. Section I deals with institutional structure of government sponsored health insurance schemes. The implementation of government sponsored health insurance schemes has been discussed in section II. Section III compares government sponsored health insurance schemes in terms of framework, coverage, benefits package, premium collection process, schemes utilisation, claims processing, hospitals network and selection of providers. Section IV concludes the whole discussion on this topic.

SECTION I

3.1 Structure of Government Sponsored Health Insurance Schemes

From the dawn of freedom, India has been trying hard to establish such universal health insurance system that would cover teeming of millions who face lack of resources. A large chunk of Indian population has remained deprived of a dependable delivery system for want of money or access to healthcare system or other constraints. Those who were in interested to frame public policies had to face the challenges of low public outlay on health about 0.9 per cent of GDP, huge unorganised labour sector i.e. 93 per cent of the labour, oversized rural members i.e. 72 per cent, freighting levels of poverty i.e. 27.5 per cent, service delivery system without any regulations and poor service of healthcare providers or hospitals increased the hurdles to the population. The policy members took keen interest in finding ways and means to reverse these trends and their efforts seems to have achieved much. Government of India's Common Minimum Programme committed itself to enhance public health outlay from 0.9 per cent to 2.2 per cent of GDP (GOI, 2004). The twelfth five-year plan (2012–17) proposals clearly highlight these issues (Planning Commission, 2011). At the same time, the products which enhance the benefit coverage are offered by the insurance industry. Government of India (both State and Central governments) are busy in devising health insurance schemes to this end.

It was in late 1940s when government sponsored health insurance schemes became known. The Employees' State Insurance Scheme (ESIS) for skilled employees was started by the central government. Central Government Health Scheme (CGHS) was introduced in about 1950 which meant coverage of union employees and their families. These made way for similar provision for those employed by railways and defence department. Almost after a half century, the insurance policies appeared in the new Avtar of GSHISs. It was due to the union government commitment to the poor people. This commanded more financial support, with the results government has to design and redesign additional financial schemes for uplifting public spending on health care from 0.9 per cent to 4.5 per cent (IRDA, 2013). All these schemes were very innovative and revolutionary because these aimed at protecting millions of BPL households under National Rural Health Mission (NRHM) and Rashtriya Swasthya Bima Yojna (RSBY). The new health insurance schemes Andhra Pradesh's Rajiv Aarogyasri Scheme, Tamil Nadu's Chief Minister Kalaignar's Health Insurance Scheme, Karnataka's Vajpayee Arogyasri Scheme were initiated by state governments. On the basis of two decade long experience in health insurance sector and these GSHISs have sound foundation. The format of these schemes was based on the structure of social insurance schemes that were going on at the time and this was also influenced by range of products provided by private insurance companies. These set of new schemes offers a covered based subsidy on a limited scale for a secondary, tertiary in patient care for the BPL population. Figure 3.1 reflects the history of GSHISs and their relationships.

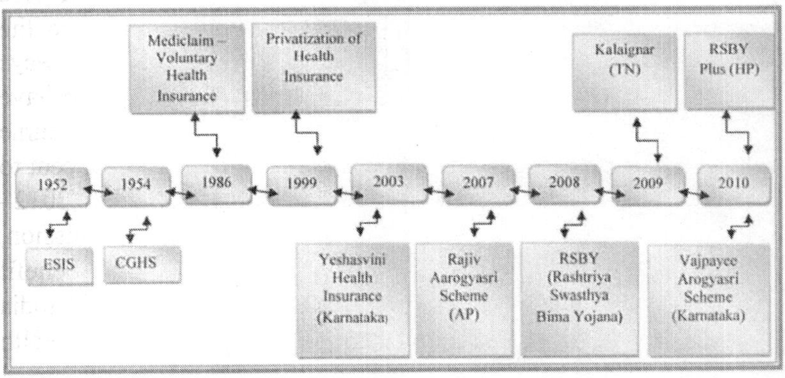

Source: GOI, 2009.

Figure 3.1: The Scenario Depicting Health Insurance Schemes in India.

3.1.1 Structure of Rashtriya Swasthya Bima Yojna (RSBY)

Ministry of Labour and Employment (MOLE) co-ordinated the functioning of RSBY and has a vital role in policy-making and implementation. The RSBY constituted to render protection huge expenditure on hospitalisation, give good quality health service access and it was ensured that the beneficiaries enjoy a choice in healthcare providers. Figure 3.1.1 displays the institutional structure of RSBY. Execution of RSBY at the national and state levels involves numerous stakeholders, the insurer being the vital link in the administration of health insurance, to empanel hospitals. Enrol beneficiaries to create

RSBY helpline and call centres in a district. Besides these, information, education and communication (IEC) activities are also to be undertaken at pre-enrollment stage and hire third-party administrators (TPAs).

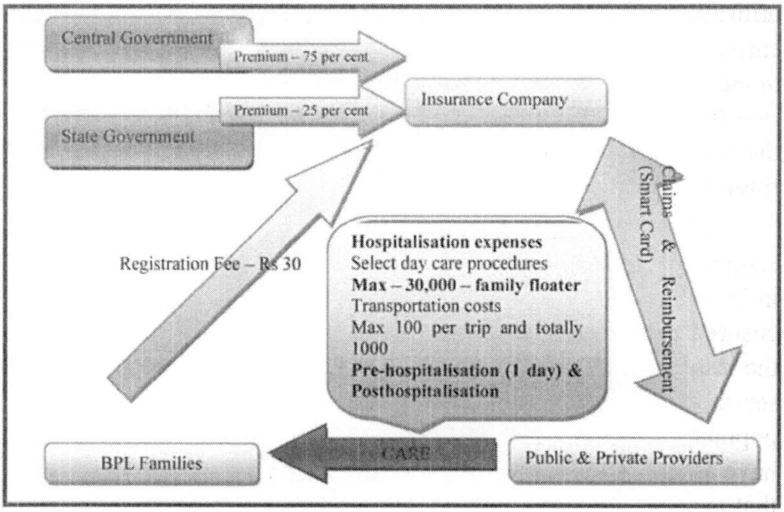

Source: Structure of RSBY obtained from www.rsby.gov.in.

Figure 3.1.1: Structure of Rashtriya Swasthya Bima Yojna (RSBY).

As and when state opts for RSBY, it has to appoint a nodal department to oversee and execute the scheme. In its turn, the concerned department establish a nodal agency to carry out the activities and execution of RSBY activities. In the process, tenders are invited from registered private and government insurance companies to decide the annual premium payable by the government per household. The lowest bidders for the technical qualification for the purpose is entrusted the job under RSBY. It is admissible for a state to invite district-wise bids if it prefers and engage different insurance companies for different states. These companies are made payment of premium on the basis of smart card issued in each district. The insurance company has to set up its office in the concerned district. There may be many insurance companies in a state providing health coverage but at one time there will be assigned all the activities on only one company in a district.

It is mandatory for the insurance company to accept the benefit package designed by MOLE in which cashless smart cards have to be made available to all the enrollees of the scheme. It has been further provided that there would be a sub-contractor to supply the eligible third party administrator and smart card provider. The insurance company will have no objection to engaging non-government organisations with local presence to act as intermediaries so that they may mobilise the BPL population for the purpose of enrollment and utilisation of after enrollment services. Thereafter hospitals are to be empanelled by the insurance companies with clear agreement for moneyless treatment. The basic minimum requirements like size and registration have to be kept in view while empanelling a hospital under the RSBY scheme. These hospitals must also make arrangements for fingerprint reader and trained staff with a special desk.

According to RSBY an enrollee is free to get treatment of his hospital of his requirement. This facility can be availed of anywhere in India from public and private hospitals. The stakeholders have been ensured of adequate incentives and benefits for their services. Since the insurance premium is based on number of household registered, it serves as a motivation for the insurance companies to cover maximum population at a extent they can reach to. In this way a hospital can have a regular flow of patients. The RSBY scheme is so lucrative so that even government hospitals would like to treat patients under the scheme because the insurer will directly pay them for the services. Many intermediaries like non-government organisations (NGOs) and micro finance institutions (MFIs) are paid for their services to the BPL population. Every biometric smart card having fingerprints and the photograph of family is issued to ensure the data flow for utilisation of services. The use of smart card is helpful in containing corruption and misuse of public money and deficiency of services, since the smart card has all Indian validity. It has become a boon for the migratory BPL population. Since treatment under RSBY involves no cash payment, the BPL beneficiaries can avail themselves of medical services and benefits upto ₹ 30,000.

3.1.2 Structure of Rajiv Aarogyasri Scheme (RAS)

The Rajiv Aarogyasri Scheme (RAS) is a health insurance scheme started by state government of Andhra Pradesh. RAS initiated for the benefit of 22.3 million BPL families for achieving healthcare. Government agencies and professional entities of Aarogyasri Health

Care Trust are the implementing agencies of the scheme. The scheme was implemented on trial basis in three districts in 2007. It was made available to all districts in a phased manner. Under the scheme a BPL household is made available a white card (Yellaiah, 2013). Coverage of expenses of up to ₹ 1.50 lakh per family per annum is ensured in hospitals. This facility can be availed by family members individually or household basis. Besides this an amount of 50,000 is also made available to cover sundry expenses. This scheme is on annual basis. Free diagnosis and treatment is done through health camps also.

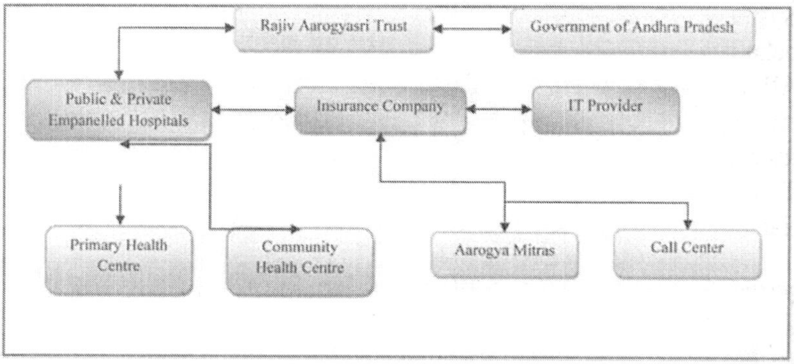

Source: Structure of RAS obtained from www.aarogyasri.org.

Figure 3.1.2: Structure of Rajiv Aarogyasri Scheme (RAS)-Andhra Pradesh.

Figure 3.1.2 shows that Rajiv Aarogyasri Trust oversees the administration of the scheme. It also takes care of fixing benefits and pricing, arranging controls with stakeholders (insurers and hospitals), meeting claims and overall monitoring. The selection of a insurance company based on open bidding process. It is the sole responsibility of insurance company to arrange health camps in villages and take treatments at their doorsteps. New members are enrolled at these camps. Star Health and Allied Insurance Company is accountable for enrolling patients, selection of hospitals and oversees the scheme. The company also selects Arogyamithra's workers at the grass root level as the first contact person for providing assistance in health insurance services to beneficiaries.

3.1.3 Structure of Chief Minister Kalaignar Health Insurance Scheme (CMKHIS)

In Tamil Nadu, Chief Minister Kaliagnar Health Insurance Scheme (CMKHIS) was introduced in 2009 to cover twenty six welfare boards and families with annual income below 72,000. The scheme based on the experience and success of RSBY. Every family gets health insurance benefits of ₹ 1 lakh extending over four years against which annual premium of ₹ 469 per family is totally given by the government of Tamil Nadu. The state health department provide funds and oversees the implementation of the scheme in the state. Tamil Nadu Health Systems Society (TNHSS) executes the health insurance scheme on behalf of the state government through the state empowered committee. Allied activities such as enrollment of beneficiaries, listing of hospitals etc. are undertaken by Star Health and Allied Insurance Company. The insurance company looks after the routine operations of the scheme. The representation of insurance company at lowest level is through liaison.

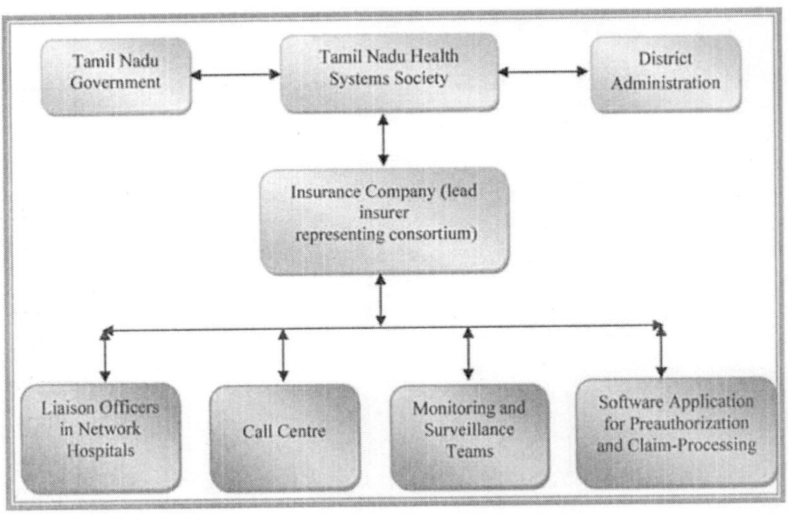

Source: Structure of CMKHIS obtained from www.tnhsp.org.

Figure 3.1.3: Structure of Chief Minister Kalaignar Health Insurance Scheme (CMKHIS) -Tamil Nadu.

3.1.4 Structure of Vajpayee Arogyasri Scheme (VAS)

Due to success and positive impact of RSBY on BPL population, Vajpayee Arogyasri Scheme (VAS) was initiated by state government of Karnataka in the year 2010. The main thrust of the scheme was to improve access of BPL population to quality healthcare, hospitalisation surgery through a network of hospitals. Six districts of Gulbarga division and two districts of Belgaum division, felt the impact of the scheme when about 3 million BPL people were connected with network of 131 hospitals, 90 per cent of which are private hospitals. The VAS provides insurer cover between ₹ 1.5 lakh to ₹ 2 lakh per family of five members for 402 procedures. Healthcare provided through the scheme is of tertiary care and is based on health camps in villages. Every hospital has to make an annual payment of ₹ 10,000 per annum to join the scheme.

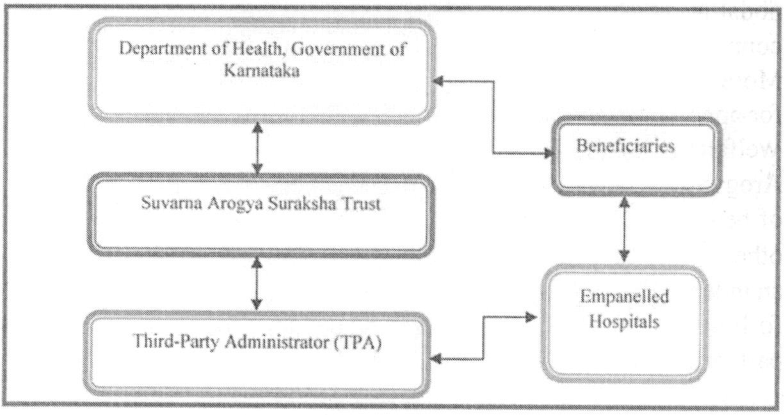

Source: Structure of VAS obtained from www.sas.gov.in.

Figure 3.1.4: Structure of Vajpayee Arogyasri Scheme (VAS) - Karnataka.

Figure 3.1.4 depicts that the Suvarna Arogya Suraksha (SAS) Trust is the decision-making body for the scheme. The routine operations are carried out by an intermediary by a three years contract. A TPA is responsible for making arrangements for hospitals and establishes a network thereof. In addition to this, the processing of claims is also undertaken by TPA. In the field, arogyamithras work as TPA's cells in hospitals. Decision-making is in the hands of an executive committee whose prior permission is a must for making any changes in design guidelines and implementation of the scheme.

SECTION II

3.2 Implementation of Government Sponsored Health Insurance Schemes

This section explains the implementing bodies of various government sponsored health insurance schemes. It explains the mechanism which is used for monitoring and evaluation of the scheme which includes registration of beneficiaries, collection of premium, distribution of resources, design and delivery of benefit package etc.

3.2.1 Implementing Agencies of GSHISs

The Table 3.2.1 depicts that at the central level, Ministry of Labour and Employment (MOLE) is the main nodal agency whose task is to see the execution of RSBY on a public-private partnership model. In the states health department, labour or rural department can serve as a nodal agency. This nodal agency is mainly looks after the activities connected with the effective and successful execution of the scheme. Moreover, the nodal agencies are suppose to arrange an open bidding for appointment of health insurers. Department of Health and Family Welfare in Karnataka has been implementing Vas from 2009. Suvarna Arogya Suraksha Trust (SAS) looks after the activities of registration of beneficiaries and making payment to concerned hospitals. On the other hand, Kalaignar health insurance scheme is being executed by an independent agency on behalf of the state government. This scheme follows the pattern of RSBY and it is based on public-private partnership model.

The implementation of the scheme is the sole responsibility of TNHSP. Since a number of insurance companies are involved in the process, Star Health and Allied Insurance Company serves as a leader and responsible for registering beneficiaries, arranging hospitals participation and settling claims under the scheme.

3.2.2 Implementation of Rashtriya Swasthya Bima Yojna (RSBY)

RSBY introduced health insurance coverage to millions of families and thousands of hospitals that had never before interacted with insurers. Early gains and recognition were helpful for the scheme to raise performance by strengthening implementation in 30 states, proper monitoring and evaluation of the scheme and minimising systemic leakage and fraud.

Table 3.2.1: Implementing Agencies

Sr. No.	*Name of the Scheme*	*Implementing Agency and Legal Status*	*Parent Department*	*Insuring Agent*	*No. of Personnel*
1.	Rashtriya Swasthya Bima Yojna (RSBY)	Ministry of Labour and Employment (MOLE) + State Nodal Agency (Society or Trust)	State Departments of Labour, Health or Rural Development	Various Insurance companies	<10 at centre + 100 at state nodal agencies
2.	Rajiv Aarogyasri Insurance Scheme (AP)	Aarogyasri Health Care Trust	Department of Health and Chief Minister's Office	STAR Health and Allied Insurance Company	117
3.	Kalaignar Health Insurance Scheme (TN)	TN Health Systems Society	Department of Health	STAR Health and Allied Insurance Company + A consortium of insurance companies	<10
4.	Vajpayee Arogyasri Scheme (KN)	Suvarna Arogya Suraksha Trust	Department of Health	Suvarna Arogya Suraksha Trust + TPA	<10

Source: Implementing agencies data obtained from www.rsby.gov.inwww.aarogyasri.org, www.tnhsp.org and www.sas.gov.in.

Table 3.2.2: State-wise Enrollment of BPL Households under RSBY

Sr. No.	States/UTs	Number of Districts		BPL Families		
		Selected	Enrollment Completed	Number of Total BPL Families	Number of BPL Families Enrolled	Take Up Ratio (in Percentage)
1.	Andhra Pradesh	1	1	2,759	2,060	74.6
2.	Arunachal Pradesh	14	10	90,312	39,615	43.8
3.	Assam	23	17	25,87,583	13,35,982	62.4
4.	Bihar	38	38	1,20,18,876	65,72,928	54.7
5.	Chandigarh	1	1	9,548	5,854	61.3
6.	Chhattisgarh	27	27	59,64,645	2,882,329	48.3
7.	Delhi	10	1	9,87,824	95,597	9.6
8.	Goa	2	2	N.A.	N.A.	N.A.
9.	Gujarat	26	26	43,70,200	17,90,585	41.0
10.	Haryana	21	21	12,63,813	4,52,045	35.8
11.	Himachal Pradesh	12	12	5,54,693	3,96,938	71.6
12.	Jammu and Kashmir	14	2	66,005	35,521	53.8
13.	Jharkhand	24	24	33,34,364	16,29,139	48.9
14.	Karnataka	30	30	40,76,642	16,76,249	41.1
15.	Kerala	14	14	3,44,6235	29,20,857	84.8
16.	Madhya Pradesh	9	2	11,10,545	3,18,314	28.7
17.	Maharashtra	32	32	45,09,135	22,64,138	50.2
18.	Manipur	6	5	1,20,237	57,995	48.2
19.	Meghalaya	11	11	4,86,695	1,99,605	40.9
20.	Mizoram	8	8	2,21,814	1,03,545	46.7

(Cond...)

21.	Nagaland	11	9	4,23,886	1,38,904	32.8
22.	Odisha	30	30	57,73,709	36,01,602	62.4
23.	Puducherry	1	1	15,142	9,486	62.6
24.	Punjab	22	22	4,53,936	1,58,517	34.9
25.	Rajasthan	33	6	36,85,055	25,83,767.	70.1
26.	Tamil Nadu	2	2	N.A.	N.A.	N.A.
27.	Tripura	7	7	7,86,913	505327	64.2
28.	Uttar Pradesh	75	75	1,10,60,686	46,53,382	42.1
29.	Uttrakhand	13	13	7,46,197	2,85,435	38.3
30.	West Bengal	19	19	96,38,922	54,24,761	56.3
	Total	**536**	**468**	**7,78,06,371**	**4,01,39,937**	**51.6**

Source: Author's calculation.

Note: Take up ratio computed from data obtained from www.rsby.gov.in as on 17th January 2014.

Note: Take up ratio is the ratio of BPL families enrolled to total BPL families.

N.A.:Data not available.

3.2.2.1 Enrollment under RSBY

Table 3.2.2 shows the extent of implementation and status of RSBY in different states of India. By the end of 2008, eleven states had enrolled under RSBY scheme, eleven more states enrolled in 2009 and by the end of 2010, four more states enrolled for Rashtriya Swasthya Bima Yojna and up to January 2014, total 30 states/UTs had enrolled under RSBY.

There were 77.80 million BPL families, out of which 40.13 million (51.6 per cent) enrolled with RSBY Scheme. 536 districts in thirty states/UTs enrolled for RSBY out of which in 468 districts enrollment had been completed and in 38 districts, it was in progress. The maximum take-up ratio of 84.8 per cent was of Kerala followed by 74.6 per cent in Andhra Pradesh. The take up ratio of Rajasthan, Chandigarh, Odisha, Tripura and Puducherry were in the range of 60-70 per cent. The take-up ratio of Bihar, Assam, Manipur, Jammu and Kashmir and Maharashtra was in the range of 50-60 per cent. The take up ratio of Gujarat, Uttar Pradesh, Jharkhand, Uttrakhand, Punjab, Haryana, Nagaland, Chhattisgarh, Meghalaya, Mizoram, Karnataka, Arunachal Pradesh and Manipur were in the range of 30-50 per cent. The minimum take up ratio 9.6 per cent was of Delhi.

3.2.2.2 Healthcare Providers under RSBY

Table 3.2.3 shows state-wise allocation of public and private healthcare providers. Beneficiaries and BPL population access healthcare benefits through any of the 11,565 empanelled hospitals spread across 536 districts, of which 7,328 (63.2 per cent) were private and 4,237 (36.8 per cent) were public hospitals.

Table 3.2.3: State-wise Distribution of Healthcare Providers

(in Numbers)

Sr. No.	*State*	*Selected Districts*	*Private Hospitals*	*Public Hospitals*	*Total Hospitals*
1.	Andhra Pradesh	1	3	4	7
2.	Arunachal Pradesh	14	-	11	11
3.	Assam	23	32	134	166
4.	Bihar	38	865	100	965
5.	Chandigarh	1	4	4	8
6.	Chhattisgarh	27	349	279	628

(Contd...)

7.	Delhi	10	35	N.A.	35
8.	Goa	2	N.A.	N.A.	N.A.
9.	Gujarat	26	937	487	1424
10.	Haryana	21	429	33	462
11.	Himachal Pradesh	12	23	171	194
12.	Jammu and Kashmir	14	5	15	20
13.	Jharkhand	24	217	220	437
14.	Karnataka	30	546	328	874
15.	Kerala	14	146	161	307
16.	Madhya Pradesh	9	76	44	120
17.	Maharashtra	32	1207	15	1222
18.	Manipur	6	6	-	6
19.	Meghalaya	11	10	188	198
20.	Mizoram	8	15	78	93
21.	Nagaland	11	6	1	7
22.	Odisha	30	137	408	545
23.	Punjab	22	175	161	336
24.	Puducherry	1	4	-	4
25.	Rajasthan	33	229	453	682
26.	Tamil Nadu	2	N.A.	N.A.	N.A.
27.	Tripura	7	1	53	54
28.	Uttar Pradesh	75	1254	730	1984
29.	Uttrakhand	13	49	94	143
30.	West Bengal	19	568	65	633
	Total	**536**	**7,328**	**4,237**	**11,565**

Source: Distribution of hospitals data computed from www.rsby.gov.in as on 17 January, 2014.
N.A.: Data not available.

The maximum hospitals were in Uttar Pradesh i.e. 1,984 of which 63.2 per cent were private hospitals and 36.8 per cent were public. Gujarat was the second leading state in which total hospitals were 1,424 of which 65.8 per cent were private and 34.2 per cent were public hospitals. May be it highlights the relationship between the government department that supervises the scheme and public health systems. There is a standard process under the scheme in respect of contact with the beneficiaries. As and when a beneficiary reaches one of the hospitals, he comes into contact with RSBY help desk whose in charge is someone from the hospital staff. Here is patient is registered and information from the smart card is downloaded. If any kind of hospitalisation is required, it is judged which package should be given to the beneficiary within the limit of ₹ 30,000. In case the requisite services not a part of the pre-defined packages, then help desk contracts the insurance company for prior-authorisation. On recovery of the patient the specific amount is determined and deducted through the smart cards. A report to this effect is transmitted to insurance company or TPA's so that reimbursement of the claim can be made. It is stipulated that claims are to be paid within the time period in 21 days, agreed upon in the contract between the insurance company and the hospital.

3.2.2.3 Utilisation and Performance of RSBY

The utilisation and performance of RSBY of three rounds are shown in Table 3.2.4. Round 1 (2008-09) consisted of 24 states (314 districts), round 2 (2009-10) consisted of 17 states (182 districts) and round 3 (2010-11) comprised 5 states (36 districts). Three rounds explain trends observed in four key performance indicators (KPIs) - claim ratio, conversion ratio, hospitalisation ratio and burnout ratio.

The average claim ratio in round one was 62.12 per cent which increased to 110.55 per cent in round 2 due to proper implementation and awareness of RSBY to BPL population and decreased to 98.79 per cent in round 3 due to lesser number of states having completed the round 3 under RSBY scheme. The average hospitalisation ratio depicts that enrollment of beneficiaries had increased during the years which showed that 1.81 per cent hospitalisation rate was in round 1, which increased to 6.05 per cent in round 3, showing positive impact of scheme on various states across India.

Table 3.2.4: Utilisation and Performance of RSBY

(in Percentage)

Sr. No.	*Round*	*States*	*Claim Ratio*	*Conversion Ratio*	*Hospitalisation Ratio*	*Expense Ratio*
1	Round 1	24	62.12	54.10	1.81	72.84
2	Round 2	17	110.55	51.18	2.64	107.26
3	Round 3	5	98.79	56.67	6.05	99.08

Source: Author's calculation.

Note: Utilisation and performance of RSBY data obtained from Ministry of Health and Family Welfare.

Note: Claim ratio is the ratio of claim paid to hospital of premium paid to insurance company minus cost of smart cards.

Note: Conversion ratio is the ratio of number of households enrolled to total number of eligible BPL families.

Note: Hospitalisation ratio is the ratio of number of hospitalisation cases to total enrollment.

Note: Expense ratio is the ratio of claim paid by insurance companies to hospital plus cost of issuance of smart cards divided by premium paid to insurance company.

The conversion ratio was 54.10 in round 1, decreased to 51.18 in round 2 and again increased to 56.67 in round 3. Large number of BPL families enrolled and availed the hospitalisation facilities. The average expense ratio in round 1 was 72.84 per cent and it was 99.08 per cent in round 3, which meant the insurance companies enjoyed the profits during the years.

3.2.2.4 Hospitalisation and Claim Ratio of RSBY

Table 3.2.5 depicts the claim and hospitalisation ratio of 24 states (314 districts), where round one had been completed. Manipur had highest claim ratio, indicating that greater number of population had been covered under the scheme. Nagaland and Delhi had claim ratio in the range of 110-120 per cent. The lowest claim ratio of 1.33 per cent was in Goa, preceded by 2.21 per cent in Assam and 2.82 per cent in Uttrakhand. Nonetheless, the average claim ratio was 62 per cent for the entire subset of states.

Table 3.2.5: State-wise Hospitalisation and Claim Ratio of RSBY in Round 1, 2 and 3

(in Percentage)

Sr. No.	*State*	*Hospitalisation Ratio*	*Claim Ratio*
1.	Assam	0.09	2.21
2.	Bihar	1.27	62.72
3.	Chandigarh	0.08	6.73
4.	Chhattisgarh	0.92	28.58
5.	Delhi	3.63	118.57
6.	Goa	0.11	1.33
7.	Gujarat	2.26	75.55
8.	Haryana	2.79	73.49
9.	Himachal Pradesh	1.70	87.33
10.	Jharkhand	0.92	42.91
11.	Karnataka	0.93	34.90
12.	Kerala	5.21	97.42
13.	Maharashtra	1.70	49.30
14.	Manipur	2.57	198.84
15.	Meghalaya	0.98	33.54
16.	Mizoram	1.75	79.29
17.	Nagaland	2.13	120.07
18.	Odisha	0.69	15.55

(Contd...)

19.	Punjab	0.95	38.26
20.	Tamil Nadu	2.62	21.42
21.	Tripura	2.69	51.40
22.	Uttar Pradesh	3.34	75.38
23.	Uttrakhand	0.76	2.82
24.	West Bengal	0.77	49.15
	Total	**1.81**	**62.12**

Source: Author's calculation.

Note: Hospitalisation and claim ratio computed from data obtained from Ministry of Health and Family Welfare.

Note: Claim ratio is the ratio of claim paid to hospital to premium paid to insurance company minus cost of smart cards.

Note: Hospitalisation ratio is the ratio of number of hospitalisation cases to total enrollment.

Assuming that enrollment, administration and allied activities amount to about 20 to 30 per cent of the premium received by the insurance companies even then they are left with some profit. It was found that hospitalisation ratio was 1.8 per cent in 24 states (314 districts) that completed round one. Kerala had highest hospitalisation ratio of 5.21 per cent and the least of 0.08 per cent was in Chandigarh. Uttar Pradesh and Delhi had hospitalisation in range of 3 -3.5 per cent. West Bengal, Uttrakhand, Punjab, Odisha, Meghalaya, Karnataka, Assam, Chhattisgarh and Goa had hospitalisation ratio of less than one per cent. The experience shows that there would be great demand for RSBY in future.

3.2.3 Implementation of Rajiv Aarogyasri Scheme (RAS)

The Rajiv Aarogyasri health insurance scheme is sponsored and funded by Andhra Pradesh for 20 million BPL families. The scheme is funded through two sources viz. regular budget of Government of Andhra Pradesh which was ₹ 925 crore funded by tax money and Chief Minister's Relief Fund (CMRF) funded by a cess on liquor which was ₹ 450 crore. The fund is pooled and managed at the level of Aarogyasri healthcare trust.

3.2.3.1 Coverage under Rajiv Aarogyasri Scheme (RAS)

Table 3.2.6 shows phase-wise coverage of Rajiv Aarogyasri Scheme. The scheme covered 198.25 lakh families out of 229.11 lakh families (86 per cent families covered) residing in 27,138 villages of 1,128 mandals of all districts of the state in five phases.

Table 3.2.6: Phase-wise Coverage under Rajiv Aarogyasri Scheme

Sr. No.	*Phase*	*Period*	*Total Families (in lakh)*	*BPL Families (in lakh)*	*Number of Procedures*	*Premium Per Family (in ₹)*
1	Phase 1	2007-08	31.12	26.67	938	489
2	Phase 2	2008-09	56.09	49.49	938	531.99
3	Phase 3	2009-10	44.30	38.44	938	489
4	Phase 4	2010-11	44.56	38.19	192	279
5	Phase 5	2011-12	53.04	45.46	192	279
	Total		**229.11**	**198.25**		

Source: BPL families and premium data obtained from annual report of Rajiv Aarogyasri scheme 2011-12.

Identification of beneficiaries was carried out through civil supplies department on the basis of ration cards. Rupees 489 is the premium amount of the scheme in phase one, which gone to ₹ 531.99 in phase two and then again decreased to ₹ 489 in phase 3. In phase 4 and 5, the premium was ₹ 279.

3.2.3.2 White-card Holders under Rajiv Aarogyasri Scheme (RAS)

Table 3.2.7 shows phase-wise issuance of white cards in Rajiv Aarogyasri scheme. The white cards had been issued to BPL families in Andhra Pradesh during five phases for providing the hospitalisation benefits to the beneficiaries.

Table 3.2.7: Phase-wise Issuance of White Cards

(in Lakhs)

Vital Statistics	*Phase I*	*Phase II*	*Phase III*	*Phase IV*	*Phase V*	*All Phases*
Population	93.35	200.66	132.91	133.67	159.12	791.71
Cards	26.28	57.33	38.45	38.19	45.46	206.11

Source: White cards data obtained from annual report of Rajiv Aarogyasri Scheme 2011-12.

A total of 206.11 lakh white cards were issued in five phases, covering 791.17 lakh beneficiaries. While 26.28 lakh cards were issued in first period, there was an abnormally high increase in phase two, when 57.33 lakh more cards had been issued to BPL people which showed awareness of the scheme among the BPL. Period III, IV and

V were also equally successful for the BPL population, when a large number of families availed themselves of the facilities.

3.2.3.3 Phase-wise Health Camps under Rajiv Aarogyasri Scheme (RAS)

The scheme was formulated in consultation with specialists from the fields of medicine, healthcare and insurance in order to address the needs of catastrophic health expenditure of the poor families of the state. The scheme is designed in such a way that the primary screening of beneficiaries is done free of charge through a system of health camps conducted at the public health care (PHC) level and also through free out-patient (OP) screening done by the network hospitals as part of scheme services. The information, education and communication (IEC) activities conducted during the health camps and OP services in network hospitals supplement the regular primary care provided by government providers.

Table 3.2.8: Phase-wise Health Camps under Rajiv Aarogyasri Scheme

(in Numbers)

Phase	*Health Camps*	*Patients Screened*	*Patients Referred*
Phase I	785	1,26,520	2,712
Phase II	1,745	2,85,770	4,654
Phase III	1,454	2,42,165	3,210
Phase IV	1,761	3,39,979	8,625
Phase V	1,738	3,34,040	10,345
Total	**7,483**	**13,28,474**	**29,546**

Source: Health camps data obtained from annual report of Rajiv Aarogyasri insurance scheme 2011-12.

Table 3.2.8 shows the phase-wise health camps, beneficiaries screened and referred under Rajiv Aarogyasri health insurance scheme. It was found that health camps had been increased from 785 in phase I to 7,483 in phase IV. There was also an increase in patients screened and referred to from 1,26,520 patients to 13,28,474 and from 2,712 patients to 29,546 patients respectively. During the year, 13.28 lakh people were screened and treated for common ailments in 7,483 health camps held under the scheme across the state. The health camps also helped in creating awareness and popularising the scheme.

3.2.3.4 Performance of the Rajiv Aarogyasri Scheme (RAS)

Table 3.2.9 shows vital statistics regarding performance of Aarogyasri health insurance scheme. Since inception of the scheme from 1st April 2007 till 27th January 2014, indicated that 36,763 check up were organised by hospitals at villages in 23 districts. Total 22,63,401 therapies operated in RAS with ratio of 27:73 of government and private.

Table 3.2.9: Performance of Rajiv Aarogyasri Scheme

Sr. No.	*Vital Statistics*	*Agency*	*Number of Health Camps*
1.	Health Camps		36,763
2.	Preauthorisation	Government	61,08,42
		Private	16,69,826
		Total	**22,80,668**
3.	Outpatients	Government	5,80,334
		Private	42,06,393
		Total	**47,86,727**
4.	Inpatient	Government	7,24,746
		Private	17,87,634
		Total	**25,12,380**
5.	Patients	Screened	73,72,401
		Registered	78,81,447
6.	Surgeries/ Therapies	Government	6,03,967
		Private	16,59,434
		Total	**22,63,401**
7.	Amount Preauthorised	Government	₹ 1,460
		Private	₹ 4,605
		Total	**₹ 6,066**
8.	Death Cases	Government	24,009
		Private	31,279
		Total	**55,288**

Source: Rajiv Aarogyasri scheme data obtained from www.aarogyasri.org as on 27th January, 2014.

There were total 25,12,380 in-patients with 28:72 ratio of government and private in-patients. There were total 47,86,727 outpatients were and the ratio of government and private out-patients was 12:88. The patients registered under the scheme were 78,81,447 from which patients screened under the scheme were 73,72,401.

Total number of therapies pre-authorised under Aarogyasri scheme were 22,80,668 and the ratio of government and private therapies pre-authorised was 27:73. Total amount pre-authorised under this scheme was ₹ 6066 crore and the ratio of government and private was 24:76. The total death cases were 55,288 and the ratio of government and private was 43:57. It was found that the private sector contributed more than the public sector and BPL population had been greatly served by the scheme.

3.2.3.5 Network Hospital Empanellment Status

Hospitals having a minimum of 50 hospital beds with requisite infrastructure and expertise within the state of Andhra Pradesh were eligible to be empanelled under the scheme for providing services. The hospitals whose applications were accepted were thereafter inducted into the scheme after a work shop and signing of agreement.

Table 3.2.10: Empanellment of Public and Private Hospitals Under RAS

(in Numbers)

Financial Year	*Public Hospitals*	*Corporate Hospitals*	*Total Hospitals*
2007-08	13	71	84
2008-09	82	207	289
2009-10	2	17	19
2010-11	0	18	18
2011-12	1	43	44
Total	**98**	**356**	**454**

Source: Network hospitals data obtained from annual report of Rajiv Aarogyasri Scheme 2011-12.

Table 3.2.10 shows empanellment of public and private hospitals under Rajiv Aarogyasri scheme from the years 2007-08 to 2011-12. There were total 454 hospitals and the ratio of public and private hospitals were 22:78 during the five phases. Maximum hospitals (289) were empanelled in the year 2008-09. The share of private hospitals was more than the public hospitals.

3.2.3.6 Therapies Preauthorised under Rajiv Aarogyasri Scheme (RAS)

The Table 3.2.11 explains that the number of surgeries pre-approved under the scheme was 17,66,119. The highest number of therapies were pre-approved in Hyderabad district (28.70 per cent), followed by Krishna district of 1,52,545 surgeries (8.63 per cent) and Visakhapatnam district of 1,51,796 surgeries (8.59 per cent). Five to nine per cent therapies were held under RAS in six districts. Lowest number of therapies 2,156 were held in Adilabad district (0.12 per cent) proceeded by Medak district of 2,357 therapies (0.13 per cent).

Table 3.2.11: District-wise Therapies Preauthorised under Rajiv Aarogyasri Scheme (RAS)

Sr. No.	*District Name*	*Number of Surgeries Preapproved*	*Percentage of Surgeries Preapproved*
1.	Hyderabad	5,06,896	28.70
2.	Adilabad	2,156	0.12
3.	Anantpur	17,875	1.01
4.	Chittoor	77,302	4.37
5.	East Godavari	1,34,251	7.60
6.	Guntur	1,45,365	8.23
7.	YSR Kadapa	10,616	0.60
8.	Khammam	16,838	0.95
9.	Kurnool	66,359	3.75
10.	Krishna	1,52,545	8.63
11.	Karimnagar	61,104	3.45
12.	Mahboobnagar	11,362	0.64
13.	Medak	2,357	0.13
14.	Nalgonda	7,824	0.44
15.	Nellore	97,306	5.50
16.	Nizamabad	14,029	0.79
17.	Prakasham	15,372	0.87
18.	Ranga Reddy	1,13,296	6.41
19.	Srikakulam	13,929	0.78
20.	Visakhapatnam	1,51,796	8.60
21.	Vizianagaram	20,643	1.16
22.	Warangal	75,066	4.25
23.	West Godavari	51,832	2.93
	Total	**17,66,119**	**100**

Source: Author's calculation.

Note: Therapies preauthorised under RAS data obtained from www.aarogyasri.org as on 2013.

3.2.4 Implementation of Chief Minister Kalaignar Health Insurance Scheme (CMKHIS)

3.2.4.1 Distribution of Smart Cards under CMKHIS

Table 3.2.12 shows that 1,29,88,796 smart cards were dispatched and 1,29,03,867 cards were distributed in Tamil Nadu in 32 districts. The highest number of smart cards 7,43,596 (5.72 per cent) were dispatched and 7,39,410 cards (5.73 per cent) distributed in Vellore.

Table 3.2.12: District-wise Distribution of Smart Cards

Sr. No.	*Districts*	*Number of Smart Cards Dispatched*	*Number of Smart Cards Distributed*	*Percentage of Smart Cards Dispatched*	*Percentage of Smart Cards Distributed*
1.	Ariyalur	1,53,243	1,53,042	1.18	1.19
2.	Chennai	4,89,530	4,72,627	3.77	3.66
3.	Coimbatore	5,97,878	5,96,116	4.60	4.62
4.	Cuddalore	5,12,126	5,04,872	3.94	3.91
5.	Dharmapuri	2,95,475	2,94,127	2.27	2.28
6.	Dindigul	3,89,550	3,87,143	3.00	3.00
7.	Erode	4,82,492	4,81,747	3.71	3.73
8.	Kancheepuram	6,41.485	6,31,364	4.94	4.89
9.	Kanyakumari	3,96,746	3,96,035	3.05	3.07
10.	Karur	2,67,880	2,67,114	2.06	2.07
11.	Krishnagiri	361,676	3,59,947	2.78	2.79
12.	Madurai	5,18,742	5,16,402	3.99	4.00
13.	Nagapattinam	2,78,609	2,78,486	2.14	2.16
14.	Namakkal	3,35,197	3,34,781	2.58	2.59
15.	Nilgiris	1,49,508	1,47,691	1.15	1.14
16.	Perambadur	1,25,500	1,24,864	0.97	0.97
17.	Pudukkattai	3,52,097	3,44,990	2.71	2.67
18.	Ramanathapuram	2,52,944	2,49,063	1.95	1.93
19.	Salem	6,26,279	6,25,266	4.82	4.85
20.	Sivagangai	2,63,114	2,60,179	2.03	2.02
21.	Thanjavur	4,79,571	4,78,702	3.69	3.71
22.	Theni	249,006	2,45,030	1.92	1.90
23.	Tirunelveli	5,23,167	5,22,760	4.03	4.05
24.	Tirupur	4,31,936	4,30,329	3.33	3.33
25.	Tiruvallur	5,38,748	5,36,848	4.15	4.16
26.	Tiruvannamalai	4,53,107	4,51,761	3.49	3.50
27.	Tiruvarur	2,81,518	2,80.340	2.17	2.17
28.	Trichy	4,91,390	4,90,333	3.78	3.80

(Cond...)

29.	Tuticorin	2,65,535	2,63,277	2.04	2.04
30.	Vellore	7,43,596	7,39,410	5.72	5.73
31.	Villupuram	7,15,486	7,15,359	5.51	5.54
32.	Virudunagar	3,25,665	3,23,862	2.51	2.51
	Total	**1,29,88,796**	**1,29,03867**	**100**	**100**

Source: Author's calculation.

Note: Distribution of smart cards data obtained from www.tnhsp.orgas on 27th January 2014.

The minimum number of smart cards 1,25,500 (0.97 per cent) were dispatched and 1,24,864 cards (0.97 per cent) were distributed in district Perambalur. The smart cards greater than five per cent dispatched and distributed in Villupuram and Vellore. Smart cards ranging between greater than three per cent but less than five per cent dispatched and distributed in fifteen districts viz. Chennai, Coimbatore, Cuddalore, Dindigul, Erode, Kancheepuram, Kanyakumari, Madurai, Salem, Thanjavur, Tirunelveli, Tirupur, Tiruvallur, Tiruvannamalai, Trichy and ten districts viz. Dharmapuri, Karur, Krishnagiri, Nagapattinam, Namakkal, Pudukkattai, Sivagangai, Tiruvarur, Tuticorin, Virudunagar were in the range of greater than two per cent but less than three per cent. Greater than one per cent but less than two per cent smart cards dispatched and distributed in Ariyalur, Theni, Ramanathapuram and Nilgiris. Perambadurs had less than one per cent of smart cards dispatched and distributed.

3.2.4.2 Enrollment of Beneficiaries under CMKHIS

Table 3.2.13 depicts the age-wise and gender-wise enrollment of beneficiaries. The total beneficiaries enrolled with Kalaignar scheme were 1,53,410 and the total premium was ₹ 41,571 lakh. The males and females ratio was 55: 45. 69,198 female beneficiaries availed the scheme contributing17,016 lakh as premium and 84,212 male beneficiaries got registered with the scheme and contributed 24,555 lakh as premium.

Female enrollment is at high level which proved that women were also known of these schemes and avail the services and shared the benefits of the schemes. However, males and females mostly of age groups 41-50 availed the benefits of this scheme. In the age group of 0-30 years, the number of males was double of females and in the age group of 91-100 years there were only 30 beneficiaries enrolled with the scheme, in which the male and female ratio was 13:87. It was

Table 3.2.13: Age-wise and Gender-wise Enrollment of Beneficiaries- 2012

Sr. No.	*Age Limit (Years)*	*Number of Females*	*Amount of Claims-Females (in ₹ lakh)*	*Number of Males*	*Amount of Claims-Males (in ₹ lakh)*	*Total Number of Beneficiaries*	*Total Amount of Claims (in ₹ lakh)*
1.	0-12	3,769	1,594	6,242	2,134	10,011	3,729
2.	13-20	3,218	1,107	6,237	1,820	9,455	2,928
3.	21-30	6,939	2,068	12,280	3,329	19,219	5,398
4.	31-40	12,601	2,982	13,839	3,810	26,440	6,792
5.	41-50	20,653	4,053	14,762	4,401	35,415	8,454
6.	51-60	13,103	3,067	14,962	4,652	28,065	7,719
7.	61-70	6,896	1,677	11,257	3,249	18,153	4,927
8.	71-80	1,770	4,058	3,983	1,004	5,753	1,410
9.	81-90	245	57	624	146	869	203
10.	91-100	4	0.82	26	5.67	30	6.49
	Total	**69,198**	**17,016**	**84,212**	**24,555**	**15,3410**	**41,571**

Source: Beneficiaries enrollment data obtained from www.tnhsp.org.

found that the beneficiaries of all the age groups from 0-100 years enjoyed the services and benefits of the scheme.

3.2.4.3 Claims and Amount Sanctioned under CMKHIS

Table 3.2.14 shows claims and amount sanctioned to various districts of Tamil Nadu under CMKHIS. There were total 1,53,410 claims with total amount of ₹ 40,648 lakh.

Table 3.2.14: Districts-wise Number of Claims and Amount Sanctioned- 2012

Sr. No.	*Districts*	*Number of Claims Approved*	*Amount (in Lakh)*	*Percentage of Claims*	*Percentage of Amount*
1.	Ariyalur	1,207	244	0.79	0.60
2.	Chennai	5,079	2,232	3.31	5.49
3.	Coimbatore	13,822	3,791	9.01	9.33
4.	Cuddalore	4,125	1,259	2.69	3.10
5.	Dharmapuri	4,030	1,218	2.63	3.00
6.	Dindigul	8,701	2,067	5.67	5.09
7.	Erode	11,740	2,600	7.65	6.40
8.	Kancheepuram	4,282	1,445	2.79	3.56
9.	Kanyakumari	6,899	1,461	4.50	3.60
10.	Karur	3,976	102	2.59	0.25
11.	Krishnagirai	3,324	1,111	2.17	2.73
12.	Madurai	4,758	1,067	3.10	2.63
13.	Negapattinam	2,855	827	1.86	2.04
14.	Namakkal	8,256	2,053	5.38	5.05
15.	Nilgiris	1,200	327	0.78	0.81
16.	Perambadur	2,417	654	1.58	1.61
17.	Pudukkattai	3,092	815	2.02	2.01
18.	Ramanathapuram	2,394	539	1.56	1.33
19.	Salem	8,860	2,547	5.78	6.27
20.	Sivagangai	2,754	610	1.80	1.50
21.	Thanjavur	5,057	1,306	3.30	3.22
22.	Theni	3,004	698	1.96	1.72
23.	Tirunelveli	3,879	985	2.53	2.43
24.	Tirupur	5,940	1,419	3.87	3.49
25.	Tiruvallur	2,347	771	1.53	1.90
26.	Tiruvannamalai	3,396	1,126	2.21	2.77
27.	Tiruvarur	2,879	759	1.88	1.87
28.	Trichy	7,340	2,038	4.78	5.02
29.	Tuticorin	2,446	561	1.59	1.38

(Cond...)

30.	Vellore	3,859	1,497	2.52	3.68
31.	Villupuram	5,452	1,680	3.55	4.14
32.	Virudunagar	4,040	819	2.63	2.02
	Total	**1,53,410**	**40,648**	**100.00**	**100.00**

Source: Author's calculation.

Note: Claims and amount sanctioned data obtained from www.tnhsp.org.

The highest number of claims 13,822 (9.01 per cent) and claim amount of ₹ 3,791 lakh (9.33 per cent) were of Coimbatore followed by 11,740 claims (7.65 per cent) and ₹ 2,600 lakh (6.40 per cent) of Erode and 8,860 claims (5.78 per cent) and ₹ 2,547 lakh (6.27 per cent) of Salem.

The least number of claims and claim amount were 1,200 claims (0.78 per cent) and ₹ 327 lakhs (0.81 per cent) of Nilgiris preceded by 1,207 claims (0.79 per cent) and ₹ 244 lakh (0.60 per cent) of Ariyalur. The amount of claims paid to beneficiaries was in the range of 4-6 per cent in five districts viz. Chennai, Dindigul, Namakkal, Tiruvarar and Nagapattinam and 2-4 per cent in fourteen districts viz. Cuddalore, Dharmapuri, Kancheepuram, Kanyakumari, Krishnagirai, Madurai, Nagapattinam, Pudukkattai, Thanjavur, Tirunelveli, Tirupur, Tiruvannamalai, Vellore and Virudunagar. The amount of claims ranging between 1-2 per cent were in six districts viz. Perambadur, Ramanathapuram, Svagangai, Theni, Tiruvallur, Tiruvarur and Tuticorin. Nilgiris and Ariyalur had claim ratio less than one per cent. The claim ratio proved that beneficiaries has utilised the scheme and availed the healthcare benefits adequately.

3.2.5 Implementation of Vajpayee Arogyasri Scheme (VAS)

3.2.5.1 Gulbarga Division Health Statistics

Table 3.2.15 shows the health camp statistics under VAS in Gulbarga division, which constituted of six districts of Karnataka namely Gulbarga, Yadagiri, Bidar, Raichur, Kopal and Bellary.

35,153 persons were enrolled in the camp and 6,738 enrollees availed the healthcare services. Eighty-two camps were held in Bellary and 7,845 persons enrolled with the scheme, out of which 1081 persons availed themselves of hospitalisation treatment.7384 persons were registered in Raichur with the scheme and 1,307 persons got treatment under the scheme. 3,182 enrollees utilised the Cardiology services,

Table 3.2.15: Gulbarga Division Health Camp Statistics- 2012

Sr. No.	*Districts*	*Camps*	*Total Registered*	*Total Referenced*	*Cardiology*	*Neuro-Surgery*	*Oncology*	*Neonatal*	*Rental*	*Polytrauma*	*Burns*
1.	Gulbarga	71	5,619	1,249	600	293	188	4	135	0	29
2.	Yadagiri	35	2,014	693	347	173	87	2	74	0	10
3.	Bidar	54	5,855	1,364	602	368	198	3	167	0	26
4.	Raichur	54	7,384	1,307	600	337	110	5	235	2	18
5.	Kopal	46	6,436	1,044	467	244	151	20	146	1	15
6.	Bellary	82	7,845	1,081	566	275	101	4	120	0	15
	Total	**342**	**3,5153**	**6,738**	**3,182**	**1,690**	**835**	**38**	**877**	**3**	**113**

Source: Health camp statistics obtained from www.sas.gov.in as on January, 2014.

followed by Neuro-surgery with 1,690 beneficiaries. Only three persons got treatment for Polytrauma. Such camps helped in creating awareness among the masses about VAS.

3.2.5.2 Claim Distribution under VAS

Table 3.2.16 shows the geographical distribution of claims across the seven districts in the Gulbarga division. There were total 3738 claims with total amount of ₹ 2197.67.

Table 3.2.16: District-wise Claim Distribution under VAS in Gulbarga Division

Sr. No.	*Districts*	*Number of Claims*	*Amount (₹ in lakh)*	*Share of Claim Value (in Per cent)*	*Average Claim Value (in ₹)*
1.	Bellary	805	486.60	22.1	60,447
2.	Bidar	658	393.05	17.9	59,734
3.	Gulbarga	931	497.17	22.6	53,402
4.	Yadagiri	350	206.93	9.4	59,124
5.	Koppal	522	319.62	14.5	61,231
6.	Raichur	464	287.39	13.1	61,938
7.	Gadag	8	6.90	0.3	86,250
	Total	**3,738**	**2,197.67**	**100.00**	**58,793**

Source: Claim distribution data obtained from Suvarna Arogya Suraksha Trust as on January, 2014.

Except Gadag, a recently created district, there were small variations in average claim values, ranging between ₹ 53,402 and ₹ 61,938. The highest numbers of cases 931 were in Gulbarga with claim value of ₹ 497.17 lakh (22.6 per cent) followed by 805 cases and claim value of ₹ 486.60 lakh (22.1 per cent) in Bellary. The variation in claim value may be the result of size of the districts and the number of beneficiary covered.

SECTION III

3.3 Comparison of Government Sponsored Health Insurance Schemes

In this section efforts have been made to compare Rashtriya Swasthya Bima Yojna (Central scheme) with other state specific public health Insurance schemes viz. Rajiv Aarogyasri scheme of Andhra Pradesh, Kalaignar Health Insurance Scheme of Tamil Nadu and Vajpayee Arogyasri Scheme of Karnataka. These schemes have been reviewed in terms of coverage, sources of finance, benefits package, premium collection process, expenditure on medical services, claims processing, revenue generation and empanellment of hospitals.

3.3.1 Flashlight on Health Insurance Coverage

Health insurance sector has received a sort of overhaul since 2007. The people benefitted from health insurance has gone up appreciably over the years under the aegis of Rashtriya Swasthya Bima Yojna, Rajiv Aarogyasri, Vajpayee Arogyasri and Kalaignar health insurance scheme taken by the union and state governments.

Table 3.3.1: Coverage under Government Sponsored Health Insurance Schemes- 2013

(in Millions)

Sr. No.	*Scheme*	*Unit of Enrollment*	*No. of Families*	*No. of Beneficiaries*	*Population*
1.	Rashtriya Swasthya Bima Yojna (RSBY)***	Family	40.13	140.45	272.3* (1270)**
2.	Rajiv Aarogyasri Scheme (RAS-AP)	Family	22.3	77.7	91.93
3.	Chief Minister Kalaignar Health Insurance Scheme (CMKHIS-TN)	Family	13.6	35	72.13
4	Vajpayee Arogyasri Scheme (VAS-KN)	Family	2.7	3.2	61.13
	Total		**78.73**	**256.35**	

Source: Coverage data obtained from www.rsby.gov.in, www.aarogyasri.org, www.tnhsp.org andwww.sas.gov.in.

* : Total BPL population in India.

** : Total population in India.

*** : RSBY data as on January, 2014.

Three of the giant schemes-Rashtriya Swasthya Bima Yojna, Rajiv Aarogyasri Scheme and Chief Minister Kalaignar Health Insurance Scheme in three years covered 185 million people in year 2010. Government sponsored health insurance schemes showed a remarkable performance in case of enrollment of beneficiaries i.e. 256.35 million from the years 2010 to 2013. Table 5.3.1 presents coverage across schemes. It was found that major enrollment is under RSBY and other state government's health insurance schemes that unitely covered 256.35 million people. By an estimate 22.3 million families and 77.7 million beneficiaries were covered in 2013 under RAS, which was about 85 per cent of the total population of the state. Kalaignar health insurance scheme covers 13.6 million families and 35 million beneficiaries, which was about 49 per cent of total population of Tamil Nadu. Vajpayee Arogyasri scheme of Karnataka covered 3.2 million beneficiaries which is about five per cent population of Karnataka. RSBY covered approximately 140.45 million individuals across the country in January, 2014 which was 52 per cent of below poverty line population in India.The coverage of RSBY is significant and vast as compared to other GSHISs and the maximum BPL population enrolled in RSBY all over country. As the coverage of RSBY is significant it has already been decided to extend the scheme beyond the BPL population. In case of state specific schemes, the coverage of RAS was also significant.

3.3.2 Sources of Finance and Mechanism Fund Policy

GSHISs revolved around collection of revenues, pooling of risk and purchasing. The source of funding mode of collecting finance and the agency involved in pooling of resources which jointly arrange financial management of the scheme.

From Table 3.3.2 it was found that the state governments pay full premium for the enrollees in three schemes-Kalaignar Health Insurance Scheme, Rajiv Aarogyasri Scheme and Vajpayee Arogyasri Scheme while 25 per cent of the premium in case of RSBY is paid by the state government and 75 per cent is paid by the central government. The premium dependents upon the type of benefit coverage.The RSBY premium payable falls in the range of ₹ 347 to ₹ 750 for a benefit cover of ₹ 30,000, whereas the premium for a cover of ₹ 2,00,000 (₹ 1,50,000 + ₹ 50,000 buffer) under Rajiv Aarogyasri scheme is ₹ 267.

The premium of Kalaignar health insurance scheme for a cover of ₹ 1,00,000 per family is ₹ 469. In case of Vajpayee Arogyasri scheme, there are no premium charges because the scheme is free.

Table 3.3.2: Sources of Finance for Government Sponsored Health Insurance Schemes

Sl. No.	*Scheme*	*Beneficiary Contribution*	*Subsidiaries (in percentage)*	*Average Premium Rates* (in ₹)*	*Coverage (in ₹)*
1.	RSBY	No	100 Centre (75) and State (25)	347 to 750	30,000 per family per year
2.	Rajiv Aarogyasri Scheme (RAS-AP)	No	100 State	267	1,50,000 per family per year with additional buffer of 50,000
3.	Kalaignar (TN)	No	100 State	N.A.	1,00,000 per family (floating over 4 years)
4.	Vajpayee Arogyasri Scheme (VAS-KN)	No	100 State	469	1,50,000 per family per year with additional buffer of 50,000

Source: Finance data obtained from www.rsby.gov.in, www.aarogyasri.org, www.tnhsp.org and www.sas.gov.in.

*: Per family per year.

N.A. : Not applicable, scheme is free.

3.3.3 Benefits and Treatment Packages

Table 3.3.3 brings out the details of healthcare and benefit packages admissible under all schemes. Moreover, it was found that coverage of all the schemes was very limited. The RSBY benefit packages mainly focus on secondary care and primary care does not form a part thereof. Chief Minister Kalaignar Health Insurance Scheme covers chronic diseases, maternity and in-patient where as Rajiv Aarogyasri Scheme and Vajpayee Arogyasri scheme only covered chronic diseases and in-patient. As compared to other schemes the scope of RSBY is very vast. Secondly healthcare services which include maternity, chronic diseases and hospitalisation are in the purview of RSBY. Though RSBY covered almost each kind of treatment yet the coverage of schemes was limited by the limit of 30,000 per family. Consequently, the packages of RSBY are used for secondary care only. On the contrary, the other schemes laid stress on tertiary healthcare including cardiovascular, cancer treatment, renal and neurological.

Table 3.3.3: Benefits and Treatment Packages under GSHISs

S. No.	*Scheme*	*Benefit Type*	*No. of Inpatient Packages*	*Coverage Extends Beyond Specified Packages*	*Maximum Annual Coverage (₹)*	*Chronic Diseases*	*Maternity*	*Preventive and Wellness Care*	*AYUSH*	*Outpatient*	*Inpatient*
1	RSBY	Inpatient Secondary Care	727	Yes	30,000/Family	✓	✓	✗	✗	✗	✓
2	Rajiv Aarogyasri (RAS-AP)	Inpatient Tertiary Care	938*	N.A.	150,000/Family+ 50,000 buffer	✓	✗	✗	✗	✗	✓
3	Kalaignar (TN)	Inpatient Tertiary Care	412	N.A.	100,000/Family (floating over 4 yrs)	✓	✓	✗	✗	✗	✓
4	Vajpayee Arogyashri (VAS-KA)	Inpatient Tertiary Care	402	N.A.	150,000/Family+ 50,000 buffer	✓	✗	✗	✗	✗	✓

Source: Benefits package data obtained from www.rsby.gov.in, www.aarogyasri.org, www.tnhsp.organd www.sas.gov.in.

*: Mostly surgical.

N.A. : Not applicable.

The schemes having maximum yearly coverage of such as RAS and VAS (coverage of ₹ 150,000/Family+ ₹ 50,000) and CMKHIS (coverage of ₹ 100,000 per household) for covered services. It was found that RSBY provides all the healthcare benefits and services within range of ₹ 30000, which is very less in comparison to other GSHISs.

Table 3.3.4: Disease Class Classified by Surgical and Medical Treatment

(in Numbers)

Sr. No.	*Various Packages*	*Surgical (S) Medical (M)*	*RSBY*	*RAS*	*CMKHIS*	*VAS*
1.	Cardiology	S	N.A.	109	24	134
		M		11	1	
2.	Nephrology	S	109	54	9	21
		M		5		
3.	Neurology	S	50	67	70	55
		M		12		
4.	Orthopaedics	S	131	68	29	8
		M		0		
5.	Gastroenterology	S	73	55	37	N.A.
		M		19		
6.	Oncology	S	23	132	121	106
		M		62	57	60
7.	Ophthalmology	S	41	26	14	
		M				N.A.
8.	Ear, Nose, and Throat (ENT)	S	71	23	3	
		M				N.A.
9.	Obstetrics and Gynaecology (OBGYN)	S	46	17	5	
		M				N.A.
10.	General Surgery	S	148	79	10	11
		M				
11.	Paediatrics	S	31	57	56	7
		M		67		
12.	Others	S	4	29	N.A.	N.A.
		M		46		
	Total		**727**	**938**	**436**	**402**
	Percentage of Surgical		**100**	**77**	**87**	**86**
	Percentage of Medical		**0**	**23**	**13**	**14**

Source: Disease group data obtained from www.rsby.gov.in, www.aarogyasri.org, www.tnhsp.org andwww.sas.gov.in.

Table 3.3.4 shows the various classes of packages by specialty. RSBY covered 727 packages in all disease groups and 100 per cent are under surgical treatment with in-patient care whereas, 938 packages are covered under Rajiv Aarogyasri Scheme with surgical and medical ratio of 77:23. Chief Minister Kalaignar Health Insurance Scheme covered 436 packages with surgical and medical ratio of 87:13 per cent and Vajpayee Arogyasri Scheme covered 402 packages with surgical and medical ratio of 86:14. Cardiology, neurosurgery, nephrology, orthopaedics, oncology, and general surgery accounted for 60 per cent of packages has been observed that the areas of paediatrics and obstetrics and gynaecology (OBGYN) possessed comparatively scantier types of treatments and procedures. In case of Nephrology, 109 packages provided under RSBY and other state sponsored schemes covered 84 packages in surgical care, whereas in case of Orthopaedics, 131 packages covered by RSBY and RAS, KHIS, VAS covered 68, 29 and 8 packages respectively. In case of Gastroenterology, Ophthalmology, Ear, Nose and Throat (ENT), Obstetrics and Gynaecology (OBGYN) and General Surgery, RSBY covered the more packages in surgery as compared to Rajiv Aarogyasri Scheme, Chief Minister Kalaignar Health Insurance Scheme and Vajpayee Arogyasri Scheme which clearly shows that RSBY provides hospitalisation services though within ₹ 30,000 as compared to other schemes.

Table 3.3.5 shows the variations in charges paid for identical packages for all procedures in different schemes and it was found that RSBY pays at a lower rate in comparison to other schemes. However, the state scheme paid more benefits on the basis of kinds of treatment in endoscopic surgery. It was seen that private care providers have charged exorbitant rates through the states due to lack of standardisation and absence of rules for them. The difference range between ₹ 30,000 to ₹ 95,000 for coronary bypass heart surgery in various schemes and it has also been found that in some cases the difference was about double.

In case of Appendectomy, RSBY covered procedures under package rate of ₹ 6,000 and RAS covered same procedures in 18,000. In case of Cholecystectomy and Hysterectomy RSBY provides the package rate of 10,000 whereas, RAS and CMKHIS provides 20,000 each. The variation ranging from 7000 to 15000 in case of

Tympanoplasty under RSBY and RAS and which showed that variation is more than double. It was found that RSBY provides the benefits and procedures under given package rates which are less than the state sponsored schemes. This clearly demonstrated that RSBY package rates cover the procedures in less amounts as compared to state sponsored schemes.

Table 3.3.5: Variation in Package Rates for Similar Procedures under GSHISs

(in ₹)

Sl. No.	*Procedure*	*RAS*	*CMKHIS*	*VAS*	*RSBY*
1.	Coronary bypass Surgery	95,000	90,000	95,000	Up to 30,000
2.	Coronary angioplasty	60,000	60,000	60,000	N.A.
3.	Transurethralresection of prostate	30,000	25,000	20,000	14,250
4.	Nephrolithotomy	10,000	25,000	10,000	10,000
5.	Nephrectomy	40,000	40,000	10,000	10,000
6.	Appendectomy	18,000	N.A.	N.A.	6,000
7.	Cholecystectomy	20,000	25,000	N.A.	10,000
8.	Hysterectomy	20,000	25,000	N.A.	10,000
9.	Tympanoplasty	15,000	N.A.	N.A.	7,000
10.	Normal delivery	N.A.	N.A.	N.A.	2,500

Source: Package rates data obtained from www.rsby.gov.in, www.aarogyasri.org, www.tnhsp.org and www.sas.gov.in.

N.A.:Not applicable.

3.3.4 Expenditure on Medical Services

Table 3.3.6 shows average central and state governments expenses of GSHISs per beneficiary and per healthcare expenditure. As far as there was high ₹ 200 per beneficiary and ₹ 60,000 per hospitalisation spending in case of Vajpayee Arogyasri Scheme. Given the state-wide rollout of the scheme, the average hospitalisation costs ₹ 28,000 and the average beneficiary cost was ₹ 180 in Rajiv Aarogyasri Scheme and in Chief Minister Kalaignar Health Insurance Scheme, the average hospitalisation costs ₹ 33,720 and the average beneficiary cost ₹ 148 which were significantly lower than those observed for Vajpayee Arogyasri. Whether it is Andhra's Aarogyasri Scheme or Tamil Nadu's Chief Minister Kalaignar Health Insurance Scheme or Karnataka's Vajpayee Arogyasri Scheme, financed by government and administered by private stakeholders, the schemes are expensive than RSBY. Secondary care is main accountability of RSBY at average cost per hospitalisation was ₹ 4,100 and per beneficiary costs were ₹ 180, which resulted that it is cheap than state health insurance schemes and shows the lowest cost per beneficiary.

Table 3.3.6: Average Government Expenses per Beneficiary per Hospitalisation

(in ₹)

Sl. No.	*Scheme*	*Per Beneficiary*	*Per Hospitalisation*
1.	RSBY*	180	4,100
2.	Rajiv Aarogyasri (AP)	171	28,000
3.	Vajpayee Arogyasri (KA)	200**	60,000**
4.	Chief Minister Kalaignar (TN)	148	33,720

Source: Beneficiary data obtained from www.rsby.gov.in, www.aarogyasri.org, www.tnhsp.org and www.sas.gov.in.

*: Estimate based on ₹ 540 average premium per family and three covered members per card.

**: Estimates are based on performance of the scheme.

RSBY covered the maximum beneficiaries with comparison of state sponsored health insurance schemes which proved that there was lowest healthcare expenditure during healthcare services. The expenditure of healthcare per beneficiary under RSBY scheme proves the tremendous administration and implementation of the scheme as compared to state sponsored schemes.

3.3.5 Processing of Claims and Use of Information Technology

During the processing of claims, in RSBY scheme the insurance company choose the TPA and this task is fulfilled by a official of a insurance company in the hospital. During the hospitalisation of BPL beneficiaries, the insurance company officials helps or supports the beneficiary for the benefits and services at hospital and ensuring the finance availability and as far as the benefits and treatment under the concerned packages. The smart card is a document required for the beneficiaries. After diagnosis of the patients and beneficiaries, when the healthcare expenses and coverage approved by concerned doctors, the expenditure of health coverage is deducted from the smart card of the covered beneficiary. The expenditure born by the health providers cleared to their account later on. The same procedure adopted under Kalaignar health insurance scheme and Vajpayee Health Insurance Scheme, where the beneficiary has to enrol in the hospital through the official of insurance company and with that procedure the patient goes through the pre-approval process. The variation between the GSHISs in case of processing of claims is only pre-approval process where the same process of diagnosis has to be informed to the insurance company through electronic media for approval. After that a group of doctors clears the claims according to services provided to the patients. The information related to post-services communicated to the insurance companies as it is mandatory step for payment of claims.

Under the government-sponsored schemes such as, Rashtriya Swasthya Bima Yojna Scheme, Chief Minister Kalaignar Health Insurance Scheme, Rajiv Aarogyasri Scheme and Vajpayee Arogyasri Scheme, smart card is being used for enrollment of the beneficiaries. The information regarding the beneficiary and his family details such as name of family members, thumb impression and photographs and balance amount for availing the healthcare services is available in the chip-based smart cards with paying a fee of ₹ 30. Free cards are provided to non-RSBY enrollees. The portability services are provided across nationwide hospitals. For settlement of claims, the insurance companies also use the smart cards for approval of packages and claims. Chief Minister Kalaignar Health Insurance Scheme, Rajiv Aarogyasri Scheme and Vajpayee Arogyasri Scheme also used chip-based smart cards for the settlement of claims.

3.3.6 Empanellment of Network Hospitals

Under the central and state sponsored health insurance schemes, the insurance company has to arrange and listing of hospitals so that the beneficiaries reap the benefits and the patients have to be treated. In this matter, there is a vital role of nodal agency for listing and selection of healthcare providers, administration of the scheme manage the hindrance during the monitoring of the performance. The ten beds are required in hospitals with fully equipped medical, surgical, diagnostic facility, qualified doctors, nursing staff, operation theatre and registration facility for the selection of healthcare providers.

Presently there were 6,121 private and 4,222 public hospitals in the network of service providers shown in Table 3.3.7. Under the Chief Minister Kalaignar Health Insurance Scheme there was a network of 692 hospitals. However, the share of public hospitals was much smaller than that of the private hospitals, there were only 56 public hospital empanelled out of 692 hospitals. In case of Rajiv Aarogyasri Scheme, the share of 77 per cent and 23 per cent were by private and public hospitals respectively.

Table 3.3.7: Number of Public and Private Hospitals Empanelled - 2013

(in Numbers)

Scheme	*Networked Hospitals*				*Total Hospitals*
	Number of Public Hospitals	*Percentage of Public Hospitals*	*Number of Private Hospitals*	*Percentage of Private Hospitals*	
RSBY*	4,237	37	7328	63	11,565
Rajiv Aarogyasri Scheme (AP)	132	23	435	77	567
Kalaignar Health Insurance Scheme (TN)	56	8	636	92	692
Vajpayee Aarogyasri Scheme (KN)'	13	10	118	90	131

Source: Hospitals data obtained from www.rsby.gov.in, www.aarogyasri.org, www.tnhsp.org and www.sas.gov.in.

*: RSBY hospitals data as on January, 2014.

It had currently 435 private and 132 government hospitals empanelled with RSBY, the number of public hospital is much higher as compared to those empanelled in Kalaignar. Vajpayee Arogyasri Scheme had more stringent criteria for empanellment of hospitals. They have been able to empanel 118 public and 13 private hospitals. The maximum numbers of hospitals i.e. 11,565 were in RSBY scheme, in which there was 63 per cent share of private hospitals and 37 per cent of public. The highest number of hospitals under RSBY scheme reveals the vast coverage and success of the scheme.

SECTION IV

3.4 Conclusion

In this chapter efforts have been made to compare the government-sponsored health insurance schemes (GSHISs) on the basis of implementation, coverage, sources of finance, benefits package, premium collection process, expenditure on medical services, claims processing, revenue generation, and selection of providers etc. GSHISs such as Rashtriya Swasthya Bima Yojna (Central scheme) and state specific initiatives include Rajiv Aarogyasri Scheme (RAS) in Andhra Pradesh, Chief Minister Kalaignar's Health Insurance Scheme (KHIS) in Tamil Nadu and Vajpayee Arogyasri Scheme (VAS) in Karnataka.

The study explained the implementation process of government sponsored health insurance schemes. Rasthriya Swasthya Bima Yojna scheme implemented in 30 states/UTs in India. There were 77.80 million BPL families out of which 40.13 million (51.6 per cent) got enrolled with RSBY Scheme. Beneficiaries could avail healthcare services from any of the 11,565 listed hospitals provides coverage in 536 districts as on January, 2014. Private hospitals made up 63 per cent (7,328 hospitals) and share of public hospitals was 37 per cent (4,237 hospitals) of the network. The Aarogyasri Health Care Trust included officials from offices of government and organisations was made accountable for the success and implementation of the Rajiv Aarogyasri scheme. White cards were given to BPL families every year, ensuring provision of the enrollees benefits. Coverage of RAS included 198.25 lakh families from which 229.11 lakh families (86 per cent families covered) living in 27,138 of the state in five Periods. Tamil Nadu Health Systems Society (TNHSS) administered the Chief Minister Kalaignar health insurance scheme. 1,29,88,796 smart cards were dispatched and 1,29,03,867 cards were distributed in Tamil Nadu. 7,43,596 (5.72 per cent) was highest number of cards dispatched and 7,39,410 cards (5.73 per cent) distributed in Vellore. According to age-wise and gender-wise, the persons registered with CMKHIS were 1,53,410 and ₹ 41,571 lakh was premium received. The ratio of male and female enrollee was 55: 45. The 69,198 female beneficiaries were registered in the scheme by giving premium of ₹ 17,016 lakh and 84,212 male beneficiaries enrolled with premium of ₹ 24555 lakh. The Suvarna Arogya Suraksha (SAS) trust looks after the activities and administration of Vajpayee Arogyasri scheme. Six districts of Gulbarga division and two districts of Belgaum division, felt the impact of the scheme when about 3 million BPL people was connected with network of 131 hospitals, 90 per cent of which are private hospitals. The VAS provides insurer cover between ₹ 1.5 lakh to ₹ 2 lakh per family of 5 members for 402 procedures.

It was found that approximately 22.3 million families were covered under RAS and 13.6 million households covering under CMKHIS. The total households under VAS are 2.2 million in 2013 and RSBY covered approximately 40.13 million BPL families nationwide in January, 2014. In comparison of government sponsored health insurance schemes, the central scheme RSBY is the one whose coverage is largest for BPL population. The totally funds/ finance provided by governments in different states for the health insurance schemes but RSBY is the scheme in which there is a responsibility of financing the scheme is of both central and states governments in the ratio of 75:25. The premium of state sponsored schemes in different states is less as compared to RSBY but in 2012 the premium charged from the companies in case of RSBY is decreased. The decrease in premium results to the fact that more and more BPL population can avail the benefits of health insurance. The scheme benefits, services and coverage are at high scale and more interesting in case of RSBY as compared to others. Rajiv Aarogyasri and Vajpayee Arogyasri Scheme only covered chronic diseases and in-patient. The comparison of government-sponsored health insurance schemes showed that RSBY provided the wide range of hospitalisation benefits to the beneficiaries across India. The motive behind the wide coverage of RSBY that five years are successfully completed and BPL population enjoys the services of all stakeholders and RSBY would extend the benefits to masses without any cost as compared to other schemes. RSBY covered mostly secondary care including maternity, chronic diseases and in-patient. In this context, health insurance schemes has a great and vital position for covering the women and reducing their problems. The extent and efficiency of health financing arrangements, the reach and performance of service delivery and the evolution of risk-protection mechanisms in India have profoundly shaped the development of government-sponsored health insurance schemes. The more organisations and infrastructure should be technologically updated for creating, designing, implementing and administering like RSBY, Rajiv Aarogyasri Scheme, Chief Minister Kalaignar Health Insurance Scheme and Vajpayee Arogyasri scheme. The implementation of government-sponsored health insurance schemes revealed that implementation has been quite successful and remarkable. RSBY provides health insurance coverage at large scale and more packages in lesser amount as compared to state specific schemes and the performance of RSBY has been quite overwhelming and upto mark.

Chapter - 4

Problems of Government Sponsored Health Insurance Schemes

In this chapter, efforts have been made to study the problems of government-sponsored health insurance schemes. The chapter is divided into three sections. Section I deals with the problems faced by government-sponsored health insurance schemes. The problems faced by the Rashtriya Swasthya Bima Yojna Scheme have been explained in section II and the whole discussion has been concluded in section III.

SECTION I

4.1 Problems of Government Sponsored Health Insurance Schemes

In this section efforts have been put to examine the characteristic problems of government-sponsored health insurance schemes and problems of Rashtriya Swasthya Bima Yojna Scheme, Rajiv Aarogyasri Scheme, Chief Minister Kalaignar Health Insurance Scheme and Vajpayee Arogyasri Scheme. The hospitalisation patterns under government-sponsored health insurance schemes and gaps in benefit coverage have also discussed in this section.

4.1.1 Characteristic Problems of Government Sponsored Health Insurance Schemes (GSHISs)

The need for medical care is unpredictable. The factors responsible for flopping of healthcare produce such a situation which leads to unethical practices, detrimental selection, fraudulent practices, malpractices besides corruption bin public health.

(1) Moral Hazard: Such a thing happens when a purchase of policy over utilises the package. Sometimes an insured indulges in such behaviour which leads to hazard to his health and more liability to the insurer. This is because of the fact that medical treatment is costly and there is great demand for medical care. However, it can operate on both fronts that is demand and supply side. Lack of authentic information between principal and agent gives a chance to the patients, health providers to reap benefits from healthcare market. In this scenario the patients tend to over utilise the facilities while the healthcare providers also realise greater gains from a wider base of patients. Whenever there is the supplier induced demand for healthcare it is always expensive and sometimes unnecessary. It has been seen that there is unnecessary treatment more than required screening, lab tests or direct overcharging.

(2) Adverse Selection: This happens when high risk patients buy insurance cover when they actually falls ill, it adds a liability to the insures simply because of lack of precautions at the time of selling the policy cover. This factor is generally more applicable to commercial schemes (Patrick *et al.,* 2010). There is sufficient proof to show that the greater difference in claims made per year for in-patient care ranges from 1.4 per cent per 1000 insured per year to more than 240 per thousand patients per year. Managers of these schemes find hard to cope with ranging claims.

(3) Malpractices and Corruption: Lack of reliable information mars the health of healthcare system. Particularly when risk pooling is through insurance in the prevalent health insurance policies, the insured, the insurance company and healthcare providers try to exploit the system as much as they can. Health providers inflate the claims with the result, they reap the higher benefits. It is so because treatment in their own hands. Data regarding various schemes suggest that the claims those were rejected differ greatly from the actual requirement. Commercial insurers have a tendency to submit fictitious claims. The rejection of claims was 16 per cent in case of commercial insurance companies while it was 4 per cent in case of RAS. However, rejection of claims was 12 per cent in respect of VAS. This was also applicable to different disease categories. The health insurance sector has seen the bogus claims to a great extent. This has been possible because detection of fraud as well as screening of every individual claim is both costly as well as manageable. With the result most of health insurance schemes are plagued by high claim ratio as well as over utilisation of facilities.

(4) Fraudulent Practices: It is interested to note that in health-care centre patients as well as hospitals connive with each other to loot the insurer. Health providers get the maximum benefits as they exploit not only the patient but also the insurance companies. It is interesting to note that with the introduction of RAS in Andhra Pradesh there have mushroomed private hospitals. Number of beds in existing hospitals has also increased phenomenally. This shows that hospitals are enjoying a regular rush of patients otherwise there would not have been a great increase in number of beds. It was estimated that bed occupancy rate is around 60 per cent while some hospitals reported to 80-110 per cent. As government envisages adding more treatment procedures the bed occupancy rate will further rise under RAS.

Another issue that state health department officials openly worry about is that their budgets may be negatively affected by the expansion of government-sponsored insurance. However, there is no evidence that public subsidies are being "converted" from the supply to the demand side. Government contributions to GSHISs appear to represent additional funds for health (Rao and Kadam, 2009). Without the presence of these schemes, it is difficult to say whether these additional funds would have been directed to public delivery or would have stayed outside the health sector itself. Also, most state schemes were created to address public supply constraints at the secondary and tertiary levels. Nevertheless, some schemes have shown intent to improve the capacity of public provision beyond what was available in the public health system. For example, schemes in Kerala and AP have provided the public hospitals with an additional source of financing that has been used to upgrade infrastructure and introduce new services (Gill, 2009).

4.1.2 The Hospitalisation Patterns under GSHISs

The government-sponsored health insurance schemes such as Rashtriya Swasthya Bima Yojna Scheme, Rajiv Aarogyasri Scheme, Chief Minister Kalaignar Health Insurance Scheme and Vajpayee Arogyasri Scheme provides only healthcare services. The big variations are found in the pattern of hospitalisation of various schemes. The comparison of packages of hospitalisation of various central and state level schemes is not according to National Sample Survey 2004. It is found that packages of hospitalisation are increased every year, which is not possible for general public to purchase the health insurance and avail the healthcare services at an increasing rate. Half of the public spending spends on tertiary health in case of Andhra Pradesh and Tamil Nadu.

Table 4.1.1: Rates of Hospitalisation in GSHISs

Scheme	*Hospitalisation per 1000 Beneficiary*	*NSSO*	
		Rural	*Urban*
Rashtriya Swasthya Bima Yojna	20	23	31
Rajiv Aarogysri Scheme (AP)	5	22	28
Chief Minister Kalaignar Health Insurance Scheme (TN)	4	23	26
Vajpayee Arogyasri Scheme (KN)	4	37	37

Source: Hospitalisation data obtained from www.rsby.gov.in, www.aarogyasri.org, www.tnhsp.org and www.sas.gov.in, NSSO Report No. 507.

Table 4.1.1 shows hospitalisation rates in government-sponsored health insurance schemes. The health schemes of different states like RAS in Andhra Pradesh, the hospitalisation rate is five per thousand whereas according to NSSO data it was 23 and 31 per 1,000 beneficiaries for rural and urban areas respectively. It was four per thousand in case of Tamil Nadu's Chief Minister Kalaignar Health Insurance Scheme which is also less than rural and urban hospitalisation rates i.e. 22 and 28 per thousand respectively. The hospitalisation rate of Karnataka's Vajpayee Arogyasri scheme is four per thousand which shows very less rates than rural and urban hospitalisation i.e. 37 per thousand in both cases. The state-based healthcare package rates are less as compared to average of Rashtriya Swasthya Bima Yojna. The reason behinds this is RSBY covered the BPL population under secondary care and dealt with routine diseases at regular rate and RAS and CMKHIS covers only uncommon diseases not at regular intervals.

4.1.3 Gaps in Benefit Coverage

According to data from NSSO (60th round), five of the top ten disease groups leading to hospitalisation for rural residents are mostly covered in the state schemes: heart disease (including hypertension), diseases of the kidney and urinary systems, gynaecological disorders, and accidents and injuries. These disease groups account for 25 per cent of admissions. Since these are generally higher-cost groups, they actually account for a still greater proportion in terms of inpatient costs. However, high-frequency but less-complex conditions such as diarrhoea, dysentery, gastritis, respiratory infections (including asthma), and malaria remain uncovered in all the state-level schemes (Gerarad and Nagpal, 2012).

These diseases are covered under RSBY. Together these groups account for 23 per cent of admissions, according to the NSSO data. Although these disease groups should ideally be treated at the primary level, an inpatient stay would represent a catastrophic expenditure for the poor. No scheme covers ambulatory care except for some initial screening of patients (e.g., at camps) to determine if their ailments merit coverage for an inpatient admission. Some schemes also have limited coverage for post-hospitalisation care (Arora and Lipika, 2011). In terms of the latter, Rashtriya Swasthya Bima Yojna (RSBY) and Rajiv Aarogyasri Scheme (RAS) cover medications for the number of days specified which are provided by the hospital upon a patient's discharge. Rajiv Aarogyasri Scheme (RAS) in Andhra Pradesh and Vajpayee Arogyasri scheme (VAS) in Karnataka also cover "follow up packages" for 125 and 50 diseases respectively. For example, in case of diseases such as renal failure and malignancies, post-hospitalisation coverage includes a year's supply of any required follow-up medicines, consultations, and defined diagnostics. These follow-up packages are, however, poorly understood and utilised.

Although these schemes reduce the financial burden for hospitalisations, whether they address the overall financial burden of the poor is an open question (Fan, 2011). Clearly, an inpatient stay would be a catastrophic event for most of the poor. For example, ambulatory care constitutes a much higher share of overall health expenditure than inpatient care and much of this continues to be out-of pocket. A chronic ailment requiring regular treatment as an out-patient can involve higher expenditures than an inpatient procedure. As schemes evolve, they will face pressure to deepen the benefits package. This has already happened in some cases. In Rajiv Aarogyasri scheme, for example, the scheme started in a small geographical area, with coverage for expensive, tertiary conditions that were among the most common causes for which patients approached the chief minister's discretionary "relief" fund for a grant to cover the cost of care (Rao, 2009). As the scheme expanded geographically, it also deepened the benefits package, adding several hundred new procedures, including some secondary procedures. Similarly, after a year of implementation experience, RSBY added maternity coverage and removed the exclusion for HIV/AIDS (Johnson and Kumar, 2011). Based on analyses of claims data, RSBY is also expanding its list of packages to standardise costs for an additional set of diseases. Also with the aim of deepening the coverage, other schemes are considering follow-up care packages. Evolution of benefits packages is an ongoing process in response to socio-political demands, claim experience, and availability of financial resources (Grover and Palacios, 2011). Given the structure of the package rates, providers have incentives to oversupply, provide additional and unnecessary care, and use treatments that maximise the coverage cap as a means to garner additional revenues from GSHISs. There is clearly a need to review rates and cost the packages in different markets, applying standardised protocols.

SECTION II

4.2 Problems of Rashtriya Swasthya Bima Yojna (RSBY)

The RSBY in its early stages of implementation achieved remarkable success in a relatively short period of time. However, it cannot be expected to address the larger problems of the health system in the short run.

4.2.1 Skewed Services by Network Hospitals

According to RSBY and other state schemes enrollment data, it has been found that there is maximum listing of private providers as compared to public. Surprisingly, on the other side the private hospitals are very less in backward areas where the need is the most. There are 63 per cent private and 37 per cent public hospitals that provided health care to RSBY beneficiaries in India in 2014.[1] It comes into light that private players covers only the creamy business and provided the services to high level customers in which case the profits are more and covers less risky ailments while referring the rest to the public healthcare. Malaria and tuberculosis do not attract their attention despite, their having serious implications for the poor. Complicated cases needing longer hospitalisation and in that cases they send the patients to government hospitals. It has been observed that there is decrease in patients as well as earnings and profits of public hospitals.

It has been stated that under RSBY scheme in Uttar Pradesh, Bihar and Gujarat, 60 per cent of hospitals put up the fraud claims. The drastic situation comes into notice that one of the districts Dangs in Gujarat state shows that without any mishappening and disease cover the false claims put up by the private hospitals. All this has been facilitated convenience with patients with help of smart cards. The claim ratio goes to 200 per cent. Sometime the hospitals claimed for households who had never been treated. The 60 hospitals have been blacklisted from the list of empanelled hospitals by Ministry of Labour.

4.2.2 Challenges Before RSBY in Earlier Stages

RSBY is the foremost central level health insurance scheme which is effectively and successfully covered the BPL population. However, RSBY scheme faced following challenges both before and during implementation:

(1) **Marketing of the Scheme:** In the early stages of RSBY scheme when it was compulsory for all the state governments. At that time it was a big challenge to convince the state governments for the RSBY officials in concerned states. The RSBY rend cooperation from all the stakeholders to create the awareness of the scheme.

(2) **Provision of Smart Card Hardware:** In the starting stages of RSBY, there was requirement of hardware to print the smart cards and distributed on the spot to number of households who were registered with the scheme. At the initiation of the scheme, there was lack of hardware, for instance smart card printer and finger print scanners. After the initiation stage, the providers of smart cards fulfilled the demand of households with the availability of hardware.

(3) **Increasing Enrollment:** In the initial stages of scheme, to enrol the BPL households was a big challenge due to incorrect date and migration of the labour class population. At that time the below poverty line population was not any information and awareness regarding the benefits of the scheme. The stakeholders such as insures and governments

of various states emerged with new ideas for instance, to increase the enrollment of BPL populations, there is a need to arrange the intermediaries such as NGOs for the information and awareness camps.

(4) **Enhancement of the Scheme:** During the early stages the utilisation of the scheme remained unknown and BPL population was not aware regarding the benefits of the scheme. It was a challenge that how smart cards serve as an indicator of the success of scheme. For providing the awareness, the insurance companies and state governments starts working jointly.

(5) **Insufficient Hospitals in Rural Areas:** There is a challenge regarding the availability of hospitals in rural and backward areas. There is huge demand which cleared that RSBY arranges the hospitals in those regions.

(6) **Capacity Development at All Levels:** To make the implementation more successful, there was a need of capacity utilisation at all levels. The challenge was proved by involving the various stakeholders at different levels. Individuals and various entities have to utilise their administrative and managerial capacities.

(7) **Standardisation:** In early period the same structure was needed for the central level scheme. All the rules and regulations, policies regarding the paper filing, smart card distribution, standardisation of software was needed to perform the similar functions at each level.

(8) **Institutional Development:** There was a requirement for central government to introduce the effective models for developing the organisational structures at the central level so that in coming periods there would be effective administration and implementation of the scheme. When that structure was organised, then its smooth running by a government entity is another task. Presently the scheme is monitored by Ministry of Labour and Family Welfare.

4.2.3 Challenges in Implementation of RSBY

The problems encountered by the RSBY were just like the problems met by such schemes around the world. The main problems can be slightly moderated but not resolved completely. But there were many such issues which called for immediate attention. This could be only done by government by stressing on the rules and their proper implementation. Sometimes the state governments did not make the payment of premium to insurance companies punctually and regularly. In some cases this method was adopted perhaps to punish the insurance companies by withholding the payments. In certain cases state governments themselves were negligent of their duties and put hurdles on the way of smooth running of the schemes. The conflict between government and insurance companies were so frequent that sometimes it became impossible to justify the programme. In some district utilisation of facilities by masses was clearly very low while the insurance companies gained heavily.

The opposite of this was also true in some cases because on an average claims ratios appeared justifiable because registration cost was sizeable. RSBY-related insurance companies had to spend ₹ 100 per household for the purpose of registrations of the household. They also had to bear the burden of service tax. Taking to account these two costs, burnout ratio was more than 80 per cent in some districts. Sometimes irritated over delayed payment of premium by governments, insurance companies went slow on making payment to hospitals.

Things aggravate in some districts to some an extent that insurance companies demanded and proposed blacklisted of some hospitals. For instance, in Dangs district of Gujarat many private hospitals had been submitted fictitious claims for months together before they were blacklisted but by that claims ratio has exceeded to 200 per cent. Small scale patients in Delhi, Kerala and Gujarat reflected the fact that 20-33 per cent, RSBY patients had to spent on medicine from their own pockets. (Nagpal, 2012).

The government-sponsored health insurance schemes are mainly funded by the government and there is almost zero contribution from the patient. In case of hospitalisation, wide variation has been observed in government-sponsored health insurance schemes (Reddy *et al.*, 2011). The hospitalisation rates of state-sponsored schemes (Rajiv Aarogyasri Scheme, Chief Minister Kalaignar Health Insurance Scheme and Vajpayee Arogyasri Scheme) were quite lower than the central scheme Rashtriya Swasthya Bima Yojna. The reason behind the variation is that state-based health insurance schemes provide for diseases which are uncommon and of comparatively little regularly. On the other hand RSBY dealt with the diseases which are common and occur regularly. With aim of deepening the coverage of health insurance, evolution of benefit packages is an ongoing process in response to socio-political demands, claim experience, and availability of financial resources.

There is a case for complementing the direct provision of health services by the government with the purchase of additional services from private providers on contractual basis. This will be more practical and desirable than relying exclusively on direct provision of health services by the government. Concerns have been often expressed about the capacity of the Ministries and Departments of Health to either directly provide healthcare services or purchase them from the private sector. The use of third parties such as insurance companies to purchase healthcare services from both the government and the private sector and to allow insured-customers to freely choose providers from whom to seek services, therefore, offers an alternative model. This has been demonstrated by the wide acceptance of insurance schemes such as the Rajiv Aarogyasri Scheme or the Rashtriya Swasthya Bima Yojna (RSBY) across several states.

4.2.4. Overcoming Challenges

The scale RSBY has been able to reach within such a short period of time is something rarely been seen in the health insurance sector across the world. It has not only been able to reach almost all the states of the country, but has also benefitted millions of people on the ground. However, there are many challenges which need to be overcome if the scheme has to be sustainable and effective in the long run. In terms of reach, the scheme should aim to cover all the intended beneficiaries who are to be subsidised by the government. To achieve this, the first priority is the preparation of a quality beneficiary data. Though the task of preparing this list lies with the other departments of the government and not with RSBY, the endeavour should be to improve the list over time, and ensure that all those who are in the list are enrolled in the scheme. Since lists of different categories are prepared by different departments/ agencies, it is critical that the de-duplication process is done on the combined list, though in the absence of common linkages between these lists it is not an easy process. Partnerships with field-based entities, which have direct access to the beneficiaries is very important and, therefore, CSOs and field-level functionaries can play a very important role in improving the lists and removing the duplicates. Similarly, once families are enrolled, it is necessary to ensure that they are not only aware of the different provisions of the scheme, but are also supported to take the benefits of the scheme through treatment at healthcare facilities. Field-level functionaries like ASHA workers, and also CSOs can play a very important role in both enrollment and hospitalisation. There have been examples in the field where organisations like the Poorest Area Civil Society (PACS) have been able to effectively reach the beneficiaries through the partner NGOs. However, this has happened only in a few states with limited number of districts. There is an urgent need to expand these initiatives to more states and districts and new partnerships needs to be formed. To leverage the existing structures at the field within the government system is also very important. Since many field-level functionaries of different departments like Auxiliary Nurse Midwives (ANMs) and ASHAs from department of health, Anganwadi workers, and village Rozgar Sevaks from rural development department are available in the field, they can be very useful in taking the message to the beneficiaries. Some states have started incentivising ASHA workers for bringing the beneficiaries to the hospitals, but much needs to be done in this regard so as to ensure that all the beneficiaries who need hospitalisation utilise the scheme. Availability of healthcare facilities, especially in the rural and remote areas is another important area which needs to be tackled. Government health facilities like community health centres (CHCs) and district hospitals are providing services, and in many states they have been able to improve their service provisions by using the RSBY claims money, yet more public health facilities need to be empanelled in all the states. In terms of private healthcare providers, though they cannot be created overnight, but the business model of RSBY is encouraging new hospitals to be set up in the remote areas. However, to sustain the interest of the private hospitals in the scheme, it is imperative that their claims are paid on time, and that there is a robust grievance redressal mechanism that is available to the hospitals in case of issues regarding empanellment or claim settlement. The state governments have set up SNAs as dedicated units to implement RSBY. From the past experience, it has been observed that the performance of the states in RSBY is dependent a lot on the strength of SNA and its capacity to implement the scheme effectively. Therefore, it is important for RSBY to build the capacities of the SNAs to effectively implement and monitor the scheme. A sum of ₹ 30 that is paid by the beneficiaries as a registration fee is used to take care of the administrative costs of the SNA. This money can be used to not only hire qualified staff for SNA, but to also carry out activities such as awareness generation, audits, etc. which help in better attainment of the scheme's objectives. Looking at the variations across states in the staffing structure of SNAs, it is important that the Government of India issues clear guidelines regarding this indicating the number and type of people required for the SNAs. One of the biggest limitations of RSBY is that it covers only in-patient treatment, while more percentage of people needs out-patient services. Almost 70 per cent of OOP expenditure on health is on out-patient and therefore, if RSBY has to achieve its objective of substantially reducing OOP expenditure on health, then it needs to include out-patient department (OPD) in its benefit package. A few experiments were initiated by the government in partnership with the private sector to provide OPD benefits to RSBY beneficiaries. Results from these experiments have shown that there is some effect on the health-seeking behaviour, and in-patient instances have come down in the districts where OPD is covered. These experiments have also demonstrated that similar technology as that of RSBY can be used to deliver OPD benefits effectively. There is a need to develop a model of providing primary care based on these experiments and experiences across the world with RSBY. If a model can be developed to link primary care, then the scheme can be much more useful in reducing OOP expenditure on health. The benefit package of RSBY is ₹ 30,000 per year for a family of five. The data of the scheme shows that only two per cent of the families have used this ₹ 30,000 out of all the families who have benefitted from the scheme. However, this can also be because the beneficiaries have not availed this scheme for costly treatment at all. Since the limit of ₹ 30,000 was set more than five years back, the government should re-look at the coverage limit. Similarly, the limit of five members may discourage enrollment of families that have more than five members. The government should increase this limit from the current five to seven members per family. Since the average enrolled family size in RSBY continues to be less than five, increasing the limit will not have much impact financially on the premium, but it will benefit such families that have more than five members. The quality of healthcare services is very important to ensure that correct treatment by qualified people is provided to the beneficiary in the time of need. However, for a large number of hospitals in India, improving the quality of care is not a priority. In the absence of any strong regulation or legal framework for ensuring quality of care, this issue becomes more complex. Experiences from other countries have shown that the quality of healthcare can be influenced through a demand-side approach. The government as a purchaser of healthcare services can influence healthcare quality strongly in the empanelled hospitals. An appropriate set of incentives and dis-incentives can be provided to the hospitals to improve their quality. Quality of care should be the priority for RSBY now, and a graded system for hospitals can be adopted for the same. Instead of creating a parallel system, efforts should be made to link it with the existing institutions like National Accreditation Board of Health (NABH) that are working on this. Issues of fraud and abuse are the most problematic areas for the insurance industry worldwide, and the RSBY too is facing this challenge. The strength of RSBY in tackling these issues lies with its data. Since data flows every day from each hospital to the government and insurance company, it can be analysed for identifying trends and patterns. There is a need to develop more scientific and robust approach to this issue. The strength in terms of availability of data can be leveraged much more than what is happening at present. The capacities of the stakeholders handling data and engaging in preventing and identifying fraud and abuse needs to be further developed.

4.2.5. Issues and Recommendations in Implementation of RSBY Scheme

Issue No. 1. Dealing with Hospital Grievances

Hospitals being the main care providers in RSBY, it is very important to have fair and transparent conditions for them from the very beginning. However, the RSBY model so far has left all dealing with hospitals to the Insurer. Insurers in turn have sub-contracted this out to Third Party Administrators (TPAs). The result is that the terms and conditions of service are left ambiguous. Since the Insurers and

TPAs have a strong incentive to contain costs, this often leads to arbitrary and unnecessary deductions in hospital bills and also delayed payments. Arbitrary treatment in turn leads to fraudulent practices on the part of hospitals.

The main complaints of hospitals against TPAs/Insurers are:

(a) Very high technology assessments used like CT, biopsy even where not strictly required. This in turn limits services provided to the larger cities.

(b) Irrational and non-transparent deductions from bills.

(c) Demand of money for processing of bills.

(d) Delayed payment of bills. Failure of TPA/Insurer to update details of pending bills in IT application.

(e) Low rates of packages. In turn this often leads to deviations on the part of hospitals.

This is a phenomenon which is reported in a study done by Amicus Advisory on RSBY. Procedures which are most commonly abused are the unspecified ward stay and ICU stay. Ward stays and ICU stays are often claimed independently of any other procedure and since no evidence is demanded, this is a common mechanism hospitals use. A study of RSBY in Amravati in Maharashtra pointed out that there was no audit of the TPA transactions and as a result inaccurate claims tended to be filed, "listing patients with ophthalmic symptoms and abdominal pain as undergoing surgical procedures, or those with fever and minor discomfort as having ICU stays". In view of all the above, a possible strategy could be to have more transparent and clearer terms of service for hospitals which are spelt out in the agreement itself. Secondly, the scope for abuse should be reduced by eliminating or re-defining packages which are abused. Finally regular monitoring of transactions should be done by State Nodal Agency by regular data collection and also through medical audit.

Recommendations on Hospital Grievances

1. Define Mandatory Investigations: These investigations should be linked to every procedure in the IT application so that hospital and insurer know what these are. These should form part of the tender and the agreement with Insurer. While laying down these investigations, it is important to keep in mind that unnecessarily technology intensive investigations should be avoided so that residents of backward areas are not discriminated against. For example, a CT scan or an ABG test is not available everywhere and should be sparingly used.

2. Lay Down Adjudication Guidelines for Claim Settlement: All insurance companies have such guidelines for claim settlement. Many such guidelines have a great deal of medical content. To ensure that good quality health protocols are built into these guidelines, these should form part of the tender and the agreement with Insurer. For instance, for orthopedic cases, these guidelines prescribe rates to be settled where more than one long bone fracture is set at the same time. These guidelines also indicate the settlement to be made where the length of stay was shorter than indicated. There are multiple such examples where each Insurer and TPA has a separate policy for settling claims for identical procedures. This in turn causes much complaint by hospitals.

3. Claims Appeal Committee should be Formed: The Insurer should be asked to set up a Claims Appeal Committee with two representatives of State Nodal Agency to entertain any appeals made by hospitals in respect of deductions and/or rejections. A turnaround time should also be prescribed for deciding on appeals. The Insurer should have final say in this matter. All hospitals need to be informed about the committee so that if needed, they can prefer appeals.

4. Draft Agreement Between Hospitals and Insurer which is Part of Rfp Should Incorporate Key Performance Indices for Hospitals for Reporting: The agreement between Hospital and Insurer which is part of the tender should contain a provision for regular reporting on Key Performance Indicators to State Nodal agency and Insurer by empanelled hospital.

5. Key Performance Indicators for Hospitals are Essential: The regular data collection is essential for being able to establish benchmarks of hospital performance on quality parameters. Such benchmarks enable assessment across time for the same facility and also across space for comparing different facilities. The data set from Maharashtra for instance collects reports on the number of admissions per month, the number of ventilator days, number of patients who left against medical advice, number of deaths, number of patients needing re-treatment for urinary stones, number of cancelled or postponed surgeries, number of surgical site infections for clean operations, other adverse events to give some example. This information would be very useful for medical audit. It is important to note that the information must be submitted on all patients treated by the hospital and not just RSBY patients. Any hospital would use substantial portions of its infrastructure to service RSBY and accordingly it should be graded on the entire infrastructure and reporting should be mandatory on outcomes for all patients.

6. Revise Hospital Rates for Packages which are Too Low as Compared to Costs: Low package rates are a common complaint by hospitals. These rates were fixed way back five years ago and cost has risen considerably since then. A committee should be appointed to work out costing of packages at current prices to fix ceiling prices afresh. A good indicator for uneconomic packages would be packages which are seldom used.

7. Initiate Medical Audit of Pre-Authorisations and Hospitals and Lay Down Strict Sanctions for Deviation: It is very important to conduct random checks by way of medical audit by the State Nodal Agency. Andhra Pradesh has done excellent work in this regard by initiating Medical audit of hospitals. For medical audit, it would be best to develop assessors from reputed medical colleges who are hired by the State Health Department for this activity. This is on the lines of the assessors on the rolls of the NABH. A third party medical audit done by a private party may not achieve much. There is a need to remember that only those doctors with sufficient standing in the medical community are capable of doing medical audit and it would be difficult for private parties to hire such people. Routinely insurers and TPAs are not able to get reputed doctors to carry out such tasks. This Medical Audit should be followed up with sanctions against hospitals which deviate from the norms. Initially the hospital concerned could be barred from performing the procedure abused but for those with many repeated offences, a recommendation regarding suspension of license under the State Nursing Homes Act could be made.

8. Re-Define Packages which are Much Abused Like Independent Ward Stay and ICU Stay: It is suggested that General ward and ICU packages should be linked with some existing packages and should not be allowed as Standalone packages. In case a patient develops a complication in an existing package prolonging length of stay indicated, only then should General Ward or ICU packages be allowed through a fresh pre-authorisation with evidence of the complication which occurred.

Issue No. 2: Running Information Technology Application

(A) No Uniformity Architecture in RSBY Currently: Currently there is no unified web based IT architecture in place in RSBY. There are two types of IT applications in RSBY: the various softwares dealing with issue of smart cards to beneficiaries and a Transaction Management Software provided by GIZ. Regarding the hospital transaction management software, there is no uniform IT application followed in RSBY across the states. SNAs have no access to the Transaction Management Software so it becomes difficult to track claim movements and settlements. This non-transparency results in piling up of complaints and grievances of network hospitals regarding claim settlements. It is therefore essential that a uniform IT application containing all the related modules, for example, preauthorisation, claims, grievances etc. should be developed and managed by the Ministry of Labour and Employment. Login rights should be given to SNAs, TPAs, Insurance Companies, network hospitals etc. per the defined requirements. Such an IT application does exist in Andhra Pradesh and Maharashtra. This web portal is a workflow-oriented integrated system which addresses the needs of all the target groups (Beneficiaries). Each phase of the patient's journey through the system, from enrollment of the beneficiary, in/out patient registration, surgery updates, preauthorisation requests, discharge updates, claim settlements etc. are routed through the IT platform. IT platform is designed for monitoring real time information about the scheme such as patients (cases) registered, preauthorisations given, surgeries performed, amount claimed by the hospitals, claim amount paid by Insurer, etc. Source code of this application could be made available to Government of India if so desired. This IT platform can be deployed at each state and it can be customizable as per the state specific requirements with minimal code changes. A provision is made in the system to add or remove procedures in the scheme. ICD coding is mandatory for all the procedures that are going to be added in to the scheme.

Data Mining: Data synchronisation/replication is very important for the MOLE to monitor the RSBY scheme progress at all the states. In order to monitor/administer the RSBY scheme centrally, IT platform should have provision for data synchronisation/replication so that all the states data (required data formats can be identified later) will be kept at one place to do any kind of analysis. This can be achieved by using interoperable techniques/Database replication techniques.

MOLE (Central RSBY) Application will enable integration of data /information from various state RSBY applications so that one-stop source for all information and data pertaining to various states can be provided to MOLE. For this purpose, patient data (RSBY cases) from various state portals need to be consolidated on a regular basis. This consolidated data will enable MOLE to monitor the scheme centrally. Approach for integrating Patient Data Replication (PDR) service with RSBY PDR service (Client) would be an integral part of State RSBY application. It is a must for consolidation of patient data from all the state RSBY portals with Central RSBY application. This can be implemented using well defined Web Service Description Language (WSDL) compliant standard interface. It provides the data of all registered patients and the data pertaining at each stage in the workflow in the given time period. This service can provide the following functionalities.

1. New patient registration

2. Patient Lifecycle updates – such as Preauthorisation, Surgery update, Claim processing, electronic health records.

3. Patient Discharge, etc.: PDR Service (server) would be an integral part of center RSBY application and it is a scheduled job type of entity. It would communicate with PDR service (client) using well defined standard interface. Using this, data can be retrieved from the state RSBY applications and kept in central database of central RSBY application.

Recommendations on IT Application

1. **Ministry of Labour Can Use Source Code of Maharashtra/ Ap Applications:** It is understood that the Ministry is already planning to have a separate agency to develop the IT application for greater functionality. Here the source code of

software as available in Maharashtra and Andhra Pradesh could be used as a basis since this software already have provisions for pre-authorisations and also for hospital claim settlement. This code could then be customized to suit RSBY.

2. **Agency for Maintaining Software should be Different from Insurer:** Once developed, this software should not be handed over for maintenance to the Insurer; rather the agency which develops the software should be hired to maintain and customize it further for a period of three years at least. Separate service level agreements could be signed between Insurers and the IT agency to facilitate data flow to the Insurer. The reasons are:

   A. **Difference in Perspective of Insurer and SNA:** All complex software require a great deal of change management and customisation. Here there is a basic conflict of interest. The Insurer is certainly interested in monitoring financial information to flag cases of fraud. But an Insurer can have no interest in the first objective of the Ministry: namely, to get epidemiological data. Capturing clinical data for this purpose requires exhaustive interaction with the users which has a cost. Insurers are rarely willing to bear these costs, nor is it in their interest to do so. Even simple activities like linking a procedure with the mandatory investigations and checklists of documents prescribed, has a cost to it.

   B. **Giving Private Insurers Control Over Health Data is Problematic:** Giving control over the IT application to the Insurer would provide private players access to the health profile of the population. That in itself is dangerous. In other countries for instance South Africa where the IT application is run by the Insurers, merely getting medical data for the government is not an easy task.

3. **Data Mining Software Needed:** Given the vast volume of data anticipated, the Ministry should invest in appropriate data mining software for retrieving data for health policy as per requirement. This data should be shared with State Nodal Agencies for appropriate action. For example, huge medical

data is available with the Arogyasri Trust in Andhra Pradesh so the Trust has incorporated a Business Intelligence tool for improved reporting, trend analysis, future projections etc. Further the invaluable data is used to study the disease trends, prevalence and distribution among various demographic groups to plan the scheme and suggest preventive health measures in AP.

Issue No. 3: Interface With Insurers

The issues discussed so far have mostly to do with implementation but we have seen that many problems also arise due to poor accountability of hospitals and insurers. The main grievance of state governments has been that the Insurers are not sufficiently accountable in the various tasks they are supposed to perform in RSBY. In this section we shall discuss the issues which arise due to errors inherent in the policy paradigm in the scheme. The basic issues in the interface with the Insurer have been:

1. Poor enrollment ratios for beneficiary families and low beneficiary awareness in many areas.
2. Skewed uptake in many regions: low uptake in some areas enables substantial profits for Insurers while fraud in other areas leads to excessive claim ratios.
3. Empanelled hospitals not equitably distributed across the region often due to concentration of hospitals in and around district headquarters and metropolises.
4. Hospitals which perform well are often de-empanelled at short notice and with little reason.
5. Medical audits are hardly conducted.
6. Information not regularly collected on Key Performance Indicators for Insurers. These issues arise mainly on account of following issues:

A. Insurance Companies are not Desgined for the Job of Outreach: Insurance companies which sell policies in the private health insurance market are not designed to conduct outreach programmes for poor and deprived beneficiaries. Private buyers are well aware of the benefits they have paid for. For group insurance policies, it is the responsibility of the company/corporation/Society to provide verified database of those eligible. In most such policies, there are routinely co-payments involved so each person covered, automatically knows the health benefits due to him. It is certainly not expected that any insurance company would make any effort to inform those covered of the benefits available. It is only with the RSBY that insurance companies were asked to make this effort. The RSBY provides coverage to the poorest and most vulnerable sections of society many of whom may not be literate. Insurance companies have little or no experience of dealing with such groups. Asking them to deliver such services has been counter-productive. A specific effort needs to be made to reach the deprived which Insurance companies do not make.

B. Conflict of Interest Over Publicity and Enrollment: Secondly, there is a major conflict of interest here. While it is true that higher enrollment would mean higher premium, too much publicity would lead to higher incidence ratios which is against the interest of the Insurer. This is why post-enrollment publicity is vested with State Nodal Agency but they have little funds for this task. Similarly empanellment of hospitals which take their tasks seriously and perform well also lead to higher payouts. De-empanellment of a hospital then cannot be so easy or at least it should not be entirely at the option of the Insurer.

C. Limited Avenues for Feedback to Government Exist: In the present RSBY structure, since the call center is run by the Insurer, very limited avenues for feedback are available to the State Nodal Agency or to the Ministry of Labour. In many states which run call centers, the average daily volume of calls is around 5000 and much information is exchanged by this means. For smooth running of the scheme, this function should be taken over by SNA.

D. Insurance Company has no Interest in Equitable Distribution of Services: Equitable distribution of facilities is a factor which is far more the concern of the State Nodal Agency than the Insurer. For insurers it hardly matters whether their payout comes from a few hospitals or from many hospitals or whether it comes from the metropolises or backward areas. This is something which does concern the State Nodal Agency which has little control over the decision. Nor are desirable ratios of beds to population spelt out in the RSBY. Since the State Nodal Agency is not sufficiently involved in these decisions, long-term plans to address basic infrastructure gaps are rarely drawn up.

E. Difference in Perspective Over it Application: From the perspective of the Insurer, the purpose of the IT application is merely to monitor the financial details of the pre-authorisations and claims and at best, to detect fraud. To add coding to capture details of medical data involves a considerable cost which is not economic from the point of view of Insurer. Given the complexity of the software, it would be very difficult to anticipate all the future requirements and build these into the Functional Requirement Specification. Moreover, while many clinical pathways exist, many are yet to be developed. Unless the IT contract is separately drawn up and monitored by the State Nodal Agency, it would be difficult to adjust the scheme to cover such requirements. In Maharashtra, the contracts which the Insurer entered into with the IT service provider ran counter to the contracts which the Insurer had signed with the State Nodal Agency.

F. Low Legitimacy for Medical Audit: Finally the ability to do medical audit depends entirely on the legitimacy of the person conducting the audit. This is something which doctors employed by Insurers rarely have. The same problem would be faced by any Third Party which attempted the task. Medical audit can best be conducted by doctors employed in reputed medical colleges or hospitals of the highest grade. Such doctors are available mostly to the government and some selected private institutes. Similarly the task of drawing up clinical pathways and lists of mandatory investigations must be coordinated by the State Nodal Agency using the services of doctors from such reputed institutions. Yet it is the Insurers who in RSBY have prescribed the lists of mandatory investigations and even on occasion, empanellment criteria.

G. Insurers cannot be Expected to Regulate Themselves: All these issues arise because of a basic anomaly in the structure of RSBY: given that the Insurer has been contracted in to perform a certain set of tasks, it must be the job of the State Nodal Agency to monitor task performance. But the RSBY creates a structure in which monitoring tasks like medical audit or grading of hospitals or collecting key performance indices from hospitals and Insurers has been entrusted to the Insurer itself. This is a contradiction in terms. No agency is equipped to regulate itself, nor should we ask it to do so. This must be the job of the State Nodal Agency. The expected outcomes and agenda must be set by the government and the State Nodal Agencies equipped with the authority and tools to monitor how that agenda could be achieved. A PPP model cannot mean outsourcing the scheme lock, stock and barrel: that would defeat the purpose of the PPP. Something like this is what has happened to the RSBY. The current allocation of tasks in RSBY does not reflect the core competence of the two main agencies involved, namely the Insurer and the State Nodal Agency. The present structure also prevents the SNA from carrying out its role of supervisor adequately. For greater efficiency and transparency in service delivery, the core competence of the agencies should be taken into account.

H. Core Competence of Insurance Companies: The core competence of an Insurance company in the field of Health Insurance lies in three main tasks:

1. Empanellment of Hospitals including fixing rates for procedures offered.
2. Processing Pre-authorisations for Elective procedures.
3. Processing Claims of Service Providers and claim settlement.

Insurers would be competent for these three tasks. However, regarding empanellment of hospitals, it is best that this should be a joint task with the State Nodal Agency. Currently empanellment is the primary responsibility of the Insurer although the State Nodal Agency can intervene where it deems fit. As has been pointed out above, it is the State Nodal Agency and not the Insurer who is interested that the hospitals be equitably distributed. Clear criteria need to be provided to the Insurer for empanellment. Also the number of hospitals in terms of ratio of bed to population should be fixed to provide some basis for decision-making. Criteria for pre-authorisation and claim settlement should also be included in the tender and also Agreement with Insurer to ensure good service and transparency. For these three tasks, Insurer does have a great deal of expertise which it may be difficult for government agencies to replicate.

I. Why State Nodal Agencies Find it Difficult to Perform the Functions of Insurer

1. **Ability of Government to Contain Costs Very Poor:** The ability of the government to keep tabs on market rates and to

negotiate discounts is severely limited. Current government procedures make any discounting of prices very difficult. The Arogyasri scheme in Andhra Pradesh started out with differential pricing for hospitals and soon after it changed to a Self-Insured Model, discounting was given up. In government hands, the likelihood is that prices of procedures would soon balloon and costs would simply remain in an upward spiral. In the Maharashtra case, the old Jeevandayee scheme processed 96000 cases at an average rate of ₹ 66000 per case for fourteen years. In the new Jeevandayee Yojna in the Insurance-based model, the cost per transaction came down to ₹ 25000 per case and the number of beneficiaries automatically tripled.

2. **Ability of Government to Manage a Varying Workload Very Poor:** Processing Pre-Authorisation and Claims is a manpower intensive task with the numbers of staff constantly varying. Given the legal hassles which all government organisations routinely face in the Labour Courts, it would be very difficult for the government to manage these aspects of the scheme. In Tamil Nadu and Maharashtra, the Insurer employs Liaison officers at every hospital, including government hospitals. Tamil Nadu insists on regular rotation of these employees. They not only facilitate patient treatment, liaison with head office but also act as informers. In Andhra Pradesh, these Arogya Mitras are employed by the Aarogyasri Trust itself and their number runs into thousands. For government however, direct employment of Arogya Mitras could have serious long-term consequences. Eventually the Arogya Mitras and the staff of the scheme would put in claims demanding permanent employment. Within six months of the scheme being launched in Maharashtra, the Arogya Mitras went on strike and only after it was made clear to them that the principal employer was the Insurer/TPA, was the strike called off.

3. **Ability of Government Agencies to Resist Political Pressures is Limited:** In India, the present political system functions on the basis of building patron-client relationships. This system in turn means that there is a great deal of

pressure on politicians from their constituents to ask for undue favours from government agencies. And hospitals are rather powerful entities. The ability of government agencies to implement empanellment norms impartially, to have an objective vetting of pre-authorisations, remains suspect therefore. Insurers on the other hand, are far less vulnerable to such pressures.

These features make insurance companies well-equipped to take care of the three tasks of empanellment, pre-authorisation and claim processing. Now let us look at the core competence of the State Nodal Agencies.

J. Core Competence of State Nodal Agency State Nodal Agencies have Long Experience in Outreach and Publicity: It has been the basic task of State governments to reach out to the public and most especially to the deprived sections of the population for the last fifty years at least. While there may have been some slip ups in the task, in the end it is government agencies which conduct the decennial census and which have built up a database of voters for the electoral machinery with some success. No doubt the databases of the government still need a great deal of correction. But that is the job of government and it cannot be outsourced. Hence the State Nodal Agency should be entrusted with the task of issuing the beneficiary cards. Given the importance of this activity, permanent kiosks could be opened for this task in the Rural Hospital in each block. The specific agencies to deliver the cards and configure each card could be empanelled by Central Government and state governments could choose any agency in the panel. It would be open to the government to pick up and empanel any competent state level public sector undertakings also for the job. Here however a note of caution is needed: the State Nodal Agencies/ concerned departments should create some paper trail involving verification by the beneficiary to validate the databases. Too often these databases are not confirmed with the beneficiary himself. Merely reading out names in a panchayat or displaying these in a ward is not sufficient to validate the databases and all caution should be taken on this account.

State Nodal Agency Well Equipped to Run Call Centre and Publicity: Most state governments already perform the task of running a call centre in the 102 service under Janani Suraksha Yojna or 108 ambulance services. So government is well up to this task. The call center is a very important source of feedback to the State Nodal Agency regarding grievances by hospitals and/or patients. Without this feedback, the ability of the State Nodal Agency to monitor the scheme becomes very limited. There are many grievances that calls are not adequately answered. All three states of Andhra Pradesh, Maharashtra and Tamil Nadu run 24×7 call centres; in AP it is done by the Aarogyasri Trust and it is run by Insurers in the other two states. Tamil Nadu supervises call center employees while the employees are paid by the Insurer. Tamil Nadu seems satisfied with the call centre but the Maharashtra government found that the information provided by the call centre staff was of varying quality ranging from good to outright bad. The Maharashtra Rajiv Gandhi Jeevandayee Arogya Yojna Society then had to set up its own call center for hospitals.

Government has Perspective Needed for Running it Application: The IT application is of great importance both for

(1) Running the scheme on a daily basis and

(2) Mining the application for health related data.

While the data gathered in RSBY has significant value, only the Health Department officials can know what the appropriate questions to ask the database are. What combination of demographic details with a particular disease pattern raises alarms is a question requiring much domain expertise. Insurance companies do not have this expertise. We should associate with reputed research institutes for data mining from the beginning; otherwise it may lose its focus in view of routine administrative works. The government should actively reach out to agencies like Indian Council of Medical Research and Medical Colleges so that the data could be used for research purposes. For all these tasks, it is important to build in fields for medical data in the various forms to be filled in by the hospitals and practitioners. Simple items like medication prescribed and ICD codes for disease and procedure, when added to demographic data, can bring in a great deal of information. This information could be used to identify any anomalies in procedures in the field and used for corrective action. Hence data mining is best possible when the state government is running the IT application. The call centre could be clubbed with the IT Application while floating a tender. Service level agreements could be drawn up between the IT vendor and Insurer. But it would be important for the SNA to directly monitor the execution of contract for the IT application.

State Nodal Agency has Access to Reputed Doctors for Conduct of Medical Audit: Conducting medical audit is an important tool to monitor the health outcomes of the scheme. The quality of treatment offered and follow up can be reviewed through audit. This task can be done by Insurers only if they have well qualified manpower. Trained doctors are not easily available to Insurers for this purpose. More importantly, in order to maintain checks and balances, it is best to have Insurers yet the pre-authorisations and claims and to have the State Nodal Agency conduct random checks both of pre-authorisations and of empanelled hospitals. The State Nodal Agency is much better equipped to conduct medical audit. The Public Health Department alone has the legitimacy required to hire doctors from reputed public and private hospitals and colleges. Finally, it is the health department alone which has an interest in and ability to monitor health outcomes.

Public Health Department has Long Experience in Working with Hospitals and Doctors: The Public Health Department has considerable experience in working with hospitals and individual doctors. It is the State Nodal agency which should identify infrastructure gaps which exist and which should draw up a long-term plan to address those gaps. Otherwise the RSBY would simply replicate the existing medical infrastructure which in turn would mean that funds would flow far more to the developed areas rather than to existing areas. Both Andhra Pradesh and Maharashtra made systematic efforts to upgrade infrastructure across the board. Maharashtra set up dialysis units in public hospitals across the state since these facilities were hardly available in the private sector. These are tasks which are of no interest to the Insurer. Only the active involvement in the empanellment process can help achieve equitable distribution in the long term.

L. Recommendations on Roles of Service Providers

Allocate Financial Functions to Insurer and Residuary Functions to State Nodal Agencies: In the light of above discussion, we can say that outsourcing the entire scheme to a single vendor would defeat the purposes of the scheme. The RSBY has some financial functions. The financial functions should rest with the Insurer but tasks like issuing of identity cards, and overall monitoring must rest with the Labour and Public Health Departments so that the health outcomes of the scheme could be monitored. For IT Application and call center, a separate vendor should be appointed to avoid conflict of interest.

Financial Functions with Insurer:

1. Processing Pre-authorisations for Elective procedures
2. Processing Claims of Service Providers and claim settlement.

For performing all these functions too, the government should provide detailed medical parameters for rationalising decision-taking in each of the above cases including clinical pathways and mandatory investigations for pre-authorisations and checklist of documents for claim processing. For processing rejected pre-authorisations more objectively, a committee consisting of two doctors from Insurer side and two doctors from SNA side could be constituted. In addition, a doctor from a public hospital mutually agreed upon by both parties, could be a fifth member. The committee would need to meet daily. Similarly a committee to process appeals on claims reduced or rejected could be constituted. Both committees should be headed by Insurer.

Supervision and Residuary Functions With SNA:

1. Issuing Smart Cards for Identification
2. Conducting Publicity
3. Conducting Medical Audits both of pre-authorisation and of hospitals and practitioners.

Joint Functions of Insurer and SNA:

1. Empanellment of Hospitals.
2. Empanellment of private practitioners for OPD services where the doctors in government or NGO sector are insufficient.

For empanellment function, a committee should be set up with two representatives of Insurer and two representatives of SNA and one representative of Public Health Department in case the SNA is the Labour Department and vice versa. The chairperson of the Empanellment Committee should be the head of the SNA.

Separate Vendor be Hired for it and Call Centre

1. Running the Call Centre

2. Running the IT Application: This tender should be separately floated by SNA and appropriate service level agreements be contracted with Insurer to facilitate scheme operations. A detailed Functional requirement specification would be needed for the tender.

Strengthen the State Nodal Agencies:

If the State Nodal Agencies are to perform all these tasks, it would be important to strengthen these agencies. Ideally each SNA should be registered as an independent society or Trust but this is a decision which should be left to the state governments. The Centre also needs to increase some resources for SNAs. Alternatively, the staff augmentation of the SNA can be done through the model followed by The Planning Commission of India, for hiring of consultants. The current allocation of ₹ 30 per family is too low and this should be raised to ₹ 50 per family insured. In any case these costs should not be loaded onto the premium. The SNA should also be provided adequate and regular training on the key processes of RSBY and the IT platform by National Labour Institute (NLI) to enable it to function effectively.

Strengthen Operations Team at MOLE: In the earlier scheme of operations, MOLE lacked the manpower to address key field issues reported to them. This was primarily done by an outsourced agency at MOLE, leaving the scheme vulnerable to multiple unresolved issues. It is hence recommended that an institutional structure be created at MOLE to support the programme at a national level. Adequate manpower at various levels technical and operational should be available at MOLE to address technical and policy level issues.

SECTION III

4.3 Conclusion

To study the problems special focus has been given to government-sponsored health insurance schemes. The government-sponsored health insurance schemes is totally free to the beneficiaries. As concerned with detrimental selection will be a concern. In such situation, the more aware purchase excessive health insurance as compared to others. This can be result of paucity of information regarding health hazards faced by the beneficiary. In healthcare, wide variation has been found in government-sponsored health insurance schemes (Nagpal, 2012).

The reason behind the variation is that state-based health insurance schemes provide high-end, rare delivery and uncommon packages, while RSBY provides largely secondary care of regular basis with common diseases. Fraud is major hindrances in the development of health insurance sector in India where the insurers are not properly followed the rules and regulations. Two kinds of frauds are there. Sometimes the insured show lack of character and submit fictitious claims. On the other hand, the hospitals themselves commit deceit on the systems.With aim of deepening the coverage of health insurance, evolution of benefit packages is an ongoing process in response to socio-political demands, claim experience, and availability of financial resources.

Rashtriya Swasthya Bima Yojna scheme faced challenges both before and during implementation. The main challenge during the implementation of the scheme was the paper and filing work of each procedure at every stage. To clear the roles and responsibility of the stakeholders is again a challenge. At every stage the stakeholders have queries regarding the bills, claims, premiums etc. In time, this trend could make the scheme unviable. Rashtriya Swasthya Bima Yojna success which is based on the effective management, administration and implementation. According to RSBY and other state schemes enrollment data, it has been found that there is maximum listing of private providers as compared to public. Surprisingly, on the other side the private hospitals are very less in backward areas where the need is the most. It has been observed that private hospitals have an increased caseload and income whereas public hospitals have shown a decline in patients, decline in the range of functions and withdrawal of funds on the assumption that income has been generated through RSBY. The government invested in primary healthcare, but the proper facilities and availability of doctors are not up to mark.

India's system of financing healthcare is full of deficiencies. To overcome these shortcomings itself is a major challenge. Situation becomes very difficult when it has to be found that masses are poor, funds are not available in enough quantities. Healthcare is beyond BPL population reach because it is very costly. It has been found that the private expenditure is three times greater the government expenditure which leads to poverty and out-of-pocket expenses. If there would increase in public health it will balance the public and private spending which will further reduces the poverty and enhance the life style of the general public.

The successful implementation of RSBY through its technology platform on a national basis and other mass-based social health insurance schemes in Andhra Pradesh, Karnataka and Tamil Nadu reflects favourably in the execution capacity and capability of health insurers. It would thus be inappropriate for the government not to harness the expertise available and act as partner with health insurers in implementation of UHC (IRDA, 2013).

Chapter - 5

Summary, Conclusion and Policy Implications

Health Insurance came into existence during the nineteenth century. The health insurance connotes a kind of insurance that makes payment for the patient's medical expenditure. Sometimes it includes coverage of disability, nursing for longer periods etc (Chahal, 2006). Such a provision is either under some government ranged programme or guaranteed by a private insurance company (Rajan and Dhunna, 2002). For any person health is of paramount importance for a person and his family. This deserves to be taken care of priority basis. Since healthy citizens make a healthy nation over a longer period of time. Insurance means reduction of financial and health risk to a every member of a group who opt for health insurance. The fund so raised from the premium of all members is utilised to compensate an unfortunate follow in the group. Insurance is such a boon which boosts an insurer's morale that an ailment cannot destabilise him economically and health-wise.

Health insurance can broadly define into four main categories – (i) Social Health Insurance; (ii) Private Health Insurance; (iii) Community Health Insurance; and (iv) Government Sponsored Health Insurance. Social health insurance (SHI) schemes are financed mainly through salaries of the employees which are based on the income or earnings. Social health insurance schemes are compulsory for the employees, workers of the particular categories. SHI Scheme is a fund organised by government with better benefits in return for contribution. It is mandatory for employees in the public and the premiums are fixed according to income but not as per the health risk.There are two social health insurance schemes first one is Central Government Health Scheme (CGHS) and the second is Employees State Insurance Scheme (ESIS). Private health insurance is a system which is optional from an insured and lucrative for the insurance companies. An insurance company is guided by profit motive and it receives premium from policyholders and make such investments to increase the insurance funds (Institute of Public Health, 2006). Community health insurance is "any not-for-profit insurance scheme that is aimed primarily at the informal sector and formed on the basis of a collective pooling of health risks and in which the members participate in its management". The government introduces a health insurance programme under government health insurance schemes (GSHISs) usually for the poorest and vulnerable sections of the community. In these schemes, the premium is totally subsidized by the government from tax-based revenues and is paid directly to the insurance company. The government introduces a health insurance programme under Government Health Insurance Schemes (GHI) usually for the below poverty population. For the BPL population, in this programme the 100 per cent financed by the government from its revenues. The important GHI schemes are (a) Rashtriya Swasthya Bima Yojna, (b) Rajiv Aarogyasri Scheme (Andhra Pradesh), (c) Chief Minister Kalaignar's Health Insurance Scheme (Tamil Nadu), (d) Vajpayee Arogyasri Scheme (PHFI, 2011).

5.1 Rationale of the Study

The study has been undertaken to examine implementation and impact of Rashtriya Swasthya Bima Yojna in India. The efforts have been also made to compare Rashtriya Swasthya Bima Yojna with other government-sponsored health insurance schemes. As the awareness and coverage of health insurance among Indian population is very less so there is a need to expand health insurance programmes to cover the population. Government has initiated various health insurance schemes for the poor and unorganised sector in India. Therefore, the present study assumes importance and the policy implications will be much useful for stakeholders, planners and policy-makers.The study will help to understand the dynamics of the health insurance both at central level as well as at the state level. The study will contribute to the body of knowledge towards examining implementation of Rashtriya Swasthya Bima Yojna and will also be helpful for the academicians, researchers and policy-makers in gaining in-depth knowledge and understanding the health insurance market in India.

Despite tremendous achievement in the health insurance sector their needs much to be done for the growth of this industry in India. Analysis of a system is a must to test it empirically to realise its importance. This study has been planned in above mentioned context. The basic objective of the study is to examine implementation and impact of Rashtriya Swasthya Bima Yojna in India. More specifically, the objectives of the study are:

(1) To work out the implementation and impact of Rashtriya Swasthya Bima Yojna in various states of India;

(2) To analyse comparative performance of Rashtriya Swasthya Bima Yojna with other public sector health insurance schemes.

(3) To study the problems faced by Government Sponsored Health Insurance Schemesin India; and

(4) To draw policy implications from the empirical analysis.

5.2 Database and Research Methodology

The present study is based on secondary data. The data used in the study were compiled primarily from World Health Organisation (WHO) reports, various monthly journals related to Rashtriya Swasthya Bima Yojna and websites etc. Further an attempt has also been made to collect the data from various organisations like Ministry of Health and Family Welfare, National Planning Commission, National Rural Health Mission, Insurance Regulatory and Development Authority, World Bank, Department of Public Health and Policy, Punjab Health Service Corporation, Employee State Insurance Corporation, Ministry of Labour and Employment, Government of India, etc.

Statistical techniques like tabular analysis, ratios, percentages, averages, coefficient of variation, pie-charts, bar-graphs etc. were applied to analyse the data for achieving the desired objectives. To identify the impact of Rashtriya Swasthya Bima Yojna on BPL population of India, the study focused on four key performance indicators (KPIs) viz. Claims Ratio (utilisation by beneficiaries), Conversion Ratio (a tool for measuring outreach), Hospitalisation Ratio (an indicator of utilisation of healthcare) and Total Expense Ratio (a parameter to judge the profit to the insurance companies).

These KPIs have been analysed from aggregated state level and insurer-wise data for the first year of operations for 24 states and 10 insurers, for the second year for 17 states and 10 insurers and for the third year for five states and four insurers.The comparison of government-sponsored health insurance schemes (GSHISs) has been analysed with the help of tabular analysis.

5.3 Implementation and Impact of Rashtriya Swasthya Bima Yojna (RSBY)

After independence Indian parliament enacted national health policy which aimed at providing health covers to masses. Health insurance scheme was amended later on in 2002. Funding of this scheme was born by Government of India and different state governments. Since the population of country is very huge the funds made by the government has always remained in sufficient for the purpose. As a result majority of Indians have to bear the cost of medical treatment for their own pockets. It is evident from National Health Accounts data that only 20 per cent of health expenditure is born by government while almost the entire amount is paid by the individuals from their own pockets. Nowhere in the world is visible is such a situation. A perusal of World Bank studies reveals that about 25 per cent of Indian population slips below the poverty line because of huge medical bills. Market for healthcare is without regulations and private health providers contributed about 77 per cent of healthcare system (Peters *et al.*, 2002). Government of India health spending has to be estimated to about 4.5 per cent of GDP while expenditure on healthcare is meagre 0.9 per cent of GDP (IRDA, 2013). Lack of funds, faulty infrastructure, low quality healthcare and poor accessibility to the rural people characterise public healthcare system.

Figures relating to rural population suggest that the highest monetary burden on the poor people's due to costly medicines and due to indoor treatment. As per estimates medicines accounted for 40 per cent of medical expenditure. Another estimate puts this figure at 75 per cent. This constituted 77 per cent for rural people and about 70 per cent for urban regions. World Health Organisation estimates suggested that in 2007, private health expenditure was about 73.5 per cent of total healthcare expenditure in India. An overwhelming amount of 90 per cent came from the pocket of concerned individuals.

Government contribution to healthcare system was just 26.5 per cent (WHO, 2010). About 94 per cent of Indian labour force is engaged with private unorganised sector. It presents a depressing spectacle that about 433 million labourers have to fend for themselves during an ailment. These people feel highly insecure because being poor they fall easy prey to illness and have to resort to medical care and treatment.The Government of India (GOI) has already made provisions of hospital insurance by subsidiary premium for the poor population. For example, in the year 2003, subsidy of ₹ 100 per family per year was paid to insurance companies for covering the population below poverty line. Universal health insurance scheme spend ₹ 1 for one person, ₹ 1.50 for a household of five members, and ₹ 2 in respect of seven members per family per day. This scheme had to be discontinued because it did not get desired response from public (Economy Watch, 2011). Therefore, in 2008, the Government of India introduced the "Rashtriya Swasthya Bima Yojna" (RSBY). RSBY is uniquely mandated to cover the entire BPL population irrespective of occupational distribution and helps to reduce out-of-pocket expenditure on healthcare and lessen a considerable financial burden on the poor. It has been an important step to supplement the efforts being made to provide quality health care to the poor and under-privileged population. It covers hospitalisation costs upto ₹ 30,000 per annum per household and scheme is jointly funded by the central and state government in the ratio of 75:25 per cent with a small contribution from the beneficiary household.The activities under the Rashtriya Swasthya Bima Yojna included the four components. Capacity Building and Information Education Communication (CBIEC), Management Information System (MIS) component, Monitoring and Evaluation (M and E) component and Institutional Development and Project Management (IDPM) component for the smooth and longer working and administration of the RSBY.

Ministry of Labour and Employment (MOLE) coordinates the scheme and lays down the policy framework. Office of the Director General–Labour Welfare plays an important role in the execution of the scheme. Making of decisions regarding format of scheme and execution there are of in the hands of MOLE. The scheme is implemented at the state level through a specially created body known as the state nodal agency (SNA). The SNA is responsible for supervision and implementation of the scheme and making arrangements with insurance companies as per the guidelines. Insurance companies are selected through bidding to participate in the bid. An insurance company must have a valid licence from the IRDA at the time of application. The insurance companies are responsible for enlisted of hospitals and make sure that their organisational structure meets scheme empanellment criteria. Insurance companies often hire third-party administrators (TPAs) to support beneficiary enrollment, hospital empanellment and claim processing services. The insurers or their TPAs may also hire smart card providers to support the enrollment process and issuing of smart cards. RSBY depends on insurance companies to a very great extent because these act as a middle person in the performance of functions of RSBY.

The RSBY characterises a successful model of symbiotic co-operation between public and private insurance companies. This is the scheme which has something for every stakeholder. Government itself feels the necessity of joining hands with private insurance companies to implement RSBY. RSBY is a scheme of the Government of India. The central Ministry of Labour defines the programme procedures, technology, data storage methods, and monitoring and evaluation, which are standardised across states.

There have been around 7.16 million hospitalisation cases from BPL families from the year 2008. In January 2014, total 30 states/ UTs have enrolled with RSBY and the total BPL families were 77.80 millions, out of which 40.13 million families (51.6 per cent) have enrolled with the RSBY. The total districts in thirty states/UT were 645 and 536 districts have enrolled for RSBY scheme out of which in 468 districts enrollment has completed and 38 districts were in progress with RSBY Scheme (www.rsby.gov.in). The take-up ratio is the ratio of BPL families enrolled divided by BPL families in selected districts. The maximum take-up ratio of 83.5 per cent was of Kerala and followed by 74.6 per cent of Arunachal Pradesh. Delhi has minimum enrollments of 9.6 per cent in RSBY Scheme. The total health care providers in RSBY were 11,565 out of which 7,328 are private and 4,237 were public hospitals. The maximum hospitals were in Uttar Pradesh i.e. 1,984 out of which 63.2 per cent were private hospitals and 36.8 per cent were public. Gujarat was the second leading state in which total hospitals were 1,424 out of which 65.8 per cent were private and 34.2 per cent were public hospitals. The maximum BPL families 19,843 have enrolled per hospital were in Nagaland as there were 86 per cent public hospitals and 14 per cent private hospitals followed by Manipur which enrolled 9,665 BPL families.The minimum BPL families 294 enrolled per hospital were in Arunachal Pradesh with ratio of 43 per cent and 57 per cent hospitals followed by 472 BPL families enrolled per hospital were in Punjab with ratio of 52 per cent private and 48 per cent public hospitals.

Efforts have been made to examine the state-wise impact of Rashtriya Swasthya Bima Yojna on below poverty line population with using claim ratio, conversion ratio, hospitalisation ratio and burnout ratio. The districts which have started implementation of RSBY in 2008 in that districts the average premium has decreased from ₹ 607 during Round 1 to ₹ 518 in Round 3, in year 2009 from ₹ 600 in round 1 to ₹ 513 in round 3, in year 2010 from ₹ 533 to ₹ 412 in round 3. This could be resulted to price correction over the years on the basis of utilisation data on large scale, increase in number of beneficiaries i.e. outreach of the scheme, decrease in cost of smart cards, installation of hardware etc. The study focused on four Key Performance Indicators (KPIs) – Claims Ratio (utilisation by beneficiaries), Conversion Ratio (a tool for measuring outreach), Hospitalisation Ratio (an indicator of utilisation of healthcare) and Total Expense Ratio (a parameter to judge profit to the insurance company). These KPIs were examined from total statewise data for the first round of 24 states (314 districts), for the second year of 17 states (182 districts) and for the third year of five states (36 districts). Ten insurance companies were participated in implementation of RSBY that completed the first round (2008-09). The same insurers continues its operations in the second round also (2009-10) and four of them again continues the scheme in third round (2010-11). This shows the positive picture of the insurance companies and their stability with the government.

Claim Ratio - In round one, the state-wise claim ratio of 24 states was 62.12 per cent which increased to 110.55 per cent in round two and it was 98.79 per cent in round three. This proved that the BPL families availed the benefits and satisfied with the services of the schemes.The state-wise comparison of claim ratio explained that in round 1, 12 states viz. Assam, Chhattisgarh, Goa, Jharkhand, Karnataka,

Maharashtra, Chandigarh, Meghalaya, Odisha, Punjab, Tamil Nadu, Uttrakhand had less than 50 per cent claim ratio, 51-100 per cent claim ratio was in nine states viz. Bihar, Gujarat, Haryana, West Bengal, Himachal Pradesh, Kerala, Mizoram, Tripura, Uttar Pradesh. Delhi and Nagaland had claim ratio in the range of 101-150 per cent and the claim ratio ranged between 151-200 per cent was only in Manipur. In round 2, the claim ratio ranged between 51-100 per cent was in nine states viz. Chhattisgarh, Delhi, Gujarat, Jharkhand, Meghalaya, Chandigarh, Nagaland, Odisha, Punjab, Uttar Pradesh, West Bengal and three states viz. Bihar, Haryana and Maharashtra, two states viz. Kerala and Uttrakhand and one state viz. Himachal Pradesh were in the range of 101-150 per cent, 151-200 per cent, 250-300 per cent respectively. This further proved that the BPL families availed the benefits and satisfied with the services and benefits of the schemes. In round 3, the highest claim ratio of 101-150 per cent was only in Uttar Pradesh and Delhi, Haryana and Kerala had claim ratio in the range of 51-100 per cent. Only Punjab had claim ratio of less than 50 per cent. From the comparison of claim ratio of three rounds, it has been found that that the second round was more beneficial to BPL families and large number of BPL families have utilised the benefits of the scheme.

The insure-wise comparison of claims ratio explained that in round one, United India Insurance Company, a public general insurer showed maximum claim ratio of 80.70 per cent and ICICI Lombard General Insurance Company, a private general insurer had highest claim ratio of 72.66 per cent, implementing greater population coverage under the scheme.In round 2, United India Insurance had highest claim ratio of 153.36 per cent followed by National Insurance Company (139.11 per cent). Tata AIG General Insurance Company, a private general insurer recorded 132.21 per cent claim ratio followed by 110.26 per cent of ICICI Lombard General Insurance Company. The increase in claim ratio resulted into increase in take up ratio among beneficiaries which further proved the positive impact of RSBY on BPL population. In round 3, Oriental Insurance Company showed highest claim ratio of 121.66 per cent and ICICI Lombard General Insurance Company showed minimum claim ratio of 64.59 per cent.

Conversion Ratio - The average conversion ratio of round one was 54.1 per cent which increased to 56.67 per cent in round 3. The increase in conversion ratio in round 3 revealed that the scheme reaches in a positive manner to BPL population and more and more BPL people registered into the scheme which availed the healthcare facilities results into enhancement of conversion. During the comparison of conversion ratio of three rounds, it has been found that in round 1, less than 20 per cent conversion ratio was observed in Assam and Delhi whereas, Mizoram, Punjab and Tamil Nadu was in the range of 21-40 per cent. The conversion ratio ranged between 41-60 per cent was in 12 states viz. Bihar, Chhattisgarh, Goa, Haryana, Jharkhand, Karnataka, Kerala, Maharashtra, Meghalaya, Odisha, Uttar Pradesh and Uttrakhand and five states viz. Gujarat, Manipur, Nagaland, West Bengal and Chandigarh have shown the conversion ratio in the range of 61-80 per cent. The maximum outreach of scheme has been shown by Himachal Pradesh and Tripura in the range of 81-100 per cent. In round 2, the significant variations have been witnessed across states. The conversion ratio of Uttar Pradesh was in the range of 21-40 per cent. Ten states viz. Bihar, Delhi, Haryana, Jharkhand, Maharashtra, Meghalaya, Odisha, Punjab, Uttrakhand and Chandigarh have shown the conversion ratio between 41-60 per cent. The conversion ratio of six states viz. Chhattisgarh, Gujarat, Himachal Pradesh, Kerala, Nagaland and West Bengal were in the range of 61-80 per cent. In round 2, the conversion ratio of RSBY was good in various states which showed the positive impact of the scheme. In round 3, Delhi has shown less than 20 per cent, Uttar Pradesh with 21-40 per cent conversion whereas; Punjab and Haryana have shown the conversion ratio in the range of 41-60 per cent. Kerala has maximum outreach of the scheme in the range of 61-80 per cent.

The comparison of insurer-wise conversion ratio showed that in round one, there were significant variations across public and private general insurers. Cholamandlam MS General Insurance Company had the highest conversion ratio of 243.30 per cent and National Insurance Company had least conversion ratio of 61.50 per cent. In second round, New India Insurance Company showed highest conversion ratio of 68.07 per cent and the least conversion ratio of 34.89 per cent was shown by Star Health. In round 3, the highest conversion ratio of 70.93 per cent was of United India Insurance and the least conversion ratio of 29.41 per cent was of Oriental Insurance Company. The increase in conversion ratio revealed that the impact of RSBY on poor people was significant while registration and utilisation was indoor treatment facilities had increased the conversion over the years.

Hospitalisation Ratio - The overall hospitalisation ratio in the first year was 1.81 per cent. It was 2.64 per cent in second year which increased to 6.05 per cent during the third year. The hospitalisation ratio in the first round proved that poor people received the benefits of the scheme to a great extent. Registration of beneficiaries when increased during the very first year hospitalisation ratio was used to find the proportion of beneficiaries via à vis the enrollment figures. This tool can be based reliably on evaluate the scheme. From the comparison of hospitalisation ratio of three rounds, it has been found that in round one, 15 states viz. Assam, Chhattisgarh, Goa, Jharkhand, Karnataka, Chandigarh, Meghalaya, Odisha, Punjab, West Bengal Uttrakhand, Bihar, Himachal Pradesh, Mizoram, Maharashtra have shown the hospitalisation ratio of less than two per cent. The hospitalisation ratio of eight states viz. Gujarat, Haryana, Manipur, Nagaland, Tamil Nadu, Tripura, Delhi and Uttar Pradesh was in the range of greater than two per cent and less than four per cent. Kerala was the only state which showed the hospitalisation ratio in the range of greater than four per cent and less than 6 per cent. The hospitalisation ratio in the first round has proved that BPL families utilised the scheme and properly availed the hospitalisation benefits. In round two, nine states viz. Nagaland, Chandigarh, Bihar, Chhattisgarh, Gujarat, Jharkhand, Meghalaya, Odisha, West Bengal have shown the hospitalisation ratio of less than two per cent and six states viz. Haryana, Maharashtra, Punjab, Uttar Pradesh, Uttrakhand and Himachal Pradesh was in the range of greater than two per cent and less than four per cent. The hospitalisation ratio of Delhi was in the range of greater than four per cent and less than six per cent and Kerala was in greater than six per cent and less than eight per cent. In third round, Punjab has shown the hospitalisation ratio of less than two per cent, Delhi, Haryana and Uttar Pradesh were in the range of greater than two per cent and less than four per cent and Kerala has shown the ratio in between greater than six per cent and less than eight per cent. The positive impact of RSBY was self-evident. Hospitalisation ratio went up to greater than six per cent and less than eight per cent during the second and third round in the states. Evidently the indoor treatment rate has been improving with the passage of time which proves that the scheme has influenced the lives of the poor people to a great extent in terms of healthcare and clearly demonstrated improvement in access to hospitalisation.

The insurer-wise comparison of hospitalisation ratio stated that United India Insurance, a public general insurer was the leading company in three rounds with highest hospitalisation ratio of 3.12 per cent, 4.63 per cent and 6.91 per cent respectively. This made United India Insurance Company the best performer during the three rounds. ICICI Lombard General Insurance Company, one private general insurer showed highest hospitalisation ratio in round 1 and two of 2.72 per cent and 3.06 per cent respectively but decrease in round 3 at 1.92 per cent due to tough competition. The comparison of hospitalisation ratios during the second and third round shows that awareness level, use of scheme and penetration there of improved considerably which is a proof of positive influence of scheme on poor people.

Burnout Ratio- The average expense ratio in round one was 72.84 per cent increased to 107.26 per cent in round two and in the third round there was a decrease in average expense ratio to 99.08 per cent. There was nominal profit in the third year. In the very first year there was an affirmative response the claimants regarding the benefits of the scheme to the poor people. The increased of hospitalisation ratio because more and more people realise the value of joining the scheme.

An analysis of burnout ratio across different rounds showed a positive trend and it has been found that the ratio is increasing over time. In round 1, the burnout ratio of seven states viz. Assam, Chhattisgarh, Goa, Odisha, Tamil Nadu, Uttrakhand and Chhandigarh was less than 50 per cent where as both the beneficiaries and the insurers were benefited. Fourteen states viz. Bihar, Gujarat, Haryana, West Bengal, Himachal Pradesh, Kerala, Mizoram, Tripura, Uttar Pradesh, Jharkhand, Karnataka, Maharashtra, Meghayala and Punjab have shown the burnout ratio ranged between 51-100 per cent. The burnout ratio of Delhi and Nagaland was in the range of 101-150 per cent whereas, Manipur was the only state ranged between 151-200 per cent. In round 2, the burnout ratio of 11 states viz. Chhattisgarh, Delhi, Gujarat, Jharkhand, Meghalaya, Chandigarh, Nagaland, Odisha, Punjab, Uttar Pradesh, West Bengal was in the range of 51-100 per cent whereas, Bihar, Haryana, Maharashtra ranged between 101-150 per cent and Kerala, Uttrakhand and Himachal Pradesh ranged between 151-200 per cent. Due to rise in the hospitalisation ratio, the burn-out ratio has increased over time. In round three, Delhi, Haryana, Kerala and Punjab have shown the burnout ratio ranged between 51-100 per cent where as only Uttar Pradesh was in range of 101-150 per cent. The burnout ratio of third round revealed that the beneficiaries have availed the hospitalisation services happily and satisfied with the scheme.

In case of insurer-wise burnout ratio in round 1, United India Insurance Company, a public general insurer had the highest burnout ratio (86.58 per cent). Among the private general insurers, ICICI Lombard General Insurance Company showed the maximum burnout ratio (80.10 per cent). It has been found that health insurance services reached to the BPL beneficiaries in a effective channel. In round two, the highest ratio was shown by United India Insurance Company (136.26 per cent) as public general insurer and Tata AIG General Insurance Company, a private general insurer showed highest burnout ratio more than 100 per cent. In round two, the burnout ratio of all the insurers increased as compared to the first round. It appeared that BPL population felt attracted towards the scheme and reaped a rich harvest of benefits provided under the RSBY. In round three, Oriental Insurance Company led with 115.28 per cent followed by United India Insurance Company (98.81 per cent). There were only four insurance companies which showed average burnout ratio of more than 100 per cent. The health insurance services were availed by the masses to great level.The trend was detrimental to the interest of insurance companies but very congenial for the welfare of the poor people.

Due to biological differences males and females encounter different health hazards. Our social norms and expectations from people add to the problem. It is fact that females generally live longer than men. Lack of resources difference in capabilities, denial of rights deprived females from healthcare. One cannot speak of health insurance for them in a traditional world. If females are provided standard health-care this can ensure them justice and equality which they need the most. With the result, enrollment of women as a percentage of total increased from 39.7 per cent in round 1 to 48.1 per cent in round 3. This shows that women were more enthusiastic about joining the RSBY. Availing of scheme also highlights the fact that women were reaping the benefits from this scheme. May be this was due to the hidden demand for healthcare in the society.

It comes into light that RSBY is giving a positive impact, as more and more BPL population registered and availing the benefits from the scheme over the time. The first round proved that poor people received the benefits of the scheme to a great extent. Registration of beneficiaries when increased during the very first year of hospitalisation ratio was used to find the proportion of beneficiaries vis-à-vis the enrollment figures. This tool can be based reliably on evaluate the scheme. The RSBY scheme is a supportive mechanism to BPL population and number of other developing countries follows this effective scheme.

5.4 Comparative Performance of Government Sponsored Health Insurance Schemes (GSHISs)

Efforts have been made to compare the government-sponsored health insurance schemes (GSHISs) on the basis of implementation, coverage, sources of finance, premium, benefit packages and empanellment of network hospitals. Before the advent of government-sponsored health insurance schemes (GSHISs), almost all public expenditure was meant for public delivery system. Since there was low public health-financing, significant responsibility issues in the system, and sizeable from the pocket expenditure by the poor patients. GSHISs came as an alternative of utilising and distribution of funds for the purpose. GSHISs have initiated a sort of new activities for administration, utilisation and management of public health resources. These changes serve as a new foundation for Indian public health delivery system. To focus on the coming issues in this sector, four GSHISs were reviewed Rashtriya Swasthya Bima Yojna (RSBY) and state specific initiatives include Rajiv Aarogyasri Scheme (RAS) in Andhra Pradesh, Chief Minister Kalaignar's Health Insurance Scheme (CMKHIS) in Tamil Nadu and Vajpayee Arogyasri Scheme (VAS) in Karnataka, so that the results obtained may be serve as guidance to all the stakeholders and policymakers.

As concerned with structure of GSHISs, Ministry of Labour and Employment (MOLE) coordinated the functioning of RSBY and has a vital role in policy-making and implementation. The RSBY constituted to render protection huge expenditure on hospitalisation, give good quality heath service access and it was ensured that the beneficiaries enjoy a choice in healthcare providers. RSBY is central scheme implemented in 2008. Central and State Governments, insurance companies, healthcare providers, beneficiaries, smart card service providers and third party administrators involved in execution of RSBY (Narayana, 2010). The Rajiv Aarogyasri Scheme (RAS) started in 2007 by state government of Andhra Pradesh. RAS initiated for the benefit BPL families for achieving healthcare. Government agencies and professional entities of Aarogyasri Health Care Trust are the implementing agencies of the scheme Yellaiah, 2013). In Tamil Nadu, Chief Minister Kalaignar Health Insurance Scheme (CMKHIS) was introduced in 2009 to cover twenty six welfare boards and families, The scheme based on the experience and success of RSBY. Allied activities such as enrollment of beneficiaries, listing of hospitals etc. are undertaken by Star Health and Allied Insurance Company. Vajpayee Arogyasri Scheme (VAS) was initiated by state government of Karnataka in the year 2010. The main thrust of the scheme was to improve access of BPL population to quality healthcare, hospitalisation surgery through a network of hospitals.

Effort has been made to explain the implementation process of government-sponsored health insurance schemes. Ministry of Labour and Employment (MOLE) is the body responsible for implementing RSBY at the central level. Rashtriya Swasthya Bima Yojna scheme has been implemented in 30 states/ UTs in India. There were 77.80 million BPL families out of which 40.13 million (51.6 per cent) got enrolled with RSBY Scheme. BPL beneficiaries can use the health insurance through any of the 11,565 empanelled hospitals spread across 536 districts as on January, 2014. Private hospitals made up 63 per cent (7,328 hospitals) and share of public hospitals was 37 per cent (4,237 hospitals) of the network. The Aarogyasri Health Care Trust constituted of government agencies and professional entities of Aarogyasri Health Care Trust which are the implementing agencies of the scheme. It was made available to all districts in a phased manner. Under the scheme a BPL household is made available a white card. The scheme covered 198.25 lakh families out of 229.11 lakh families (86 per cent families covered) residing in 27,138 villages of 1128 mandals of all districts of the state in five phases. Each year the BPL families registered with the scheme and there was a tough competition in between the insurance companies due to which the premium decreased from ₹ 489 in Phase 1 to ₹ 279 in Phase 5. Total number of therapies preauthorised under Aarogyasri scheme was 21,64,072 and the ratio of government and private therapies preauthorised was 26:74. Total amount preauthorised under this scheme was ₹ 5,747 crore, and the ratio of government and private was 24:76. The private sector contributed more than the public sector.

Tamil Nadu has entrusted the Tamil Nadu Health Systems Society (TNHSS) to implement the Chief Minister Kalaignar Health Insurance Scheme. There were 1,07,90,538 smart cards dispatched and 1,07,40,806 cards distributed in 32 districts of Tamil Nadu. The total beneficiaries enrolled with Kalaignar health insurance scheme were 1,53,410 and the total amount of premium was ₹ 41,571 lakh. The men and women ratio was 55:45. 69,198 women were enrolled by paying the amount of ₹ 17,016 lakh and 84,212 men beneficiaries registered by paying premium of ₹ 24,555 lakh (Selvavinayagam and Vijayakumar, 2012). The beneficiaries of all the age groups from 0-100 years availed the benefits of the scheme. There were total 1,53,410 claims with total amount of ₹ 40,648 lakh.

Suvarna Arogya Suraksha (SAS) Trust is the decision-making body for the scheme. The routine operations are carried out by an intermediary by a three years contract. A TPA is responsible for making arrangements for hospitals and establishes a network thereof. In addition to this, the processing of claims is also undertaken by TPA. In the field, arogyamithras work as TPA's cells in hospitals. Decision-making is in the hands of an executive committee whose prior permission is a must for making any changes in design guidelines and implementation of the scheme. The VAS has been operational in six districts of Gulbarga division and two districts of Belgaum division, with an overall 30 lakh BPL population with 131 network hospitals (90 per cent of them private). By an estimate, 2.2 million families enrolled with VAS. A health camp under VAS was held in Gulbarga division where in six districts of Karnataka participated. 35,153 persons got themselves registered in the camp and 6,738 enrollees availed hospitalisation services. These camps were helpful for creating the awareness among the BPL population. There were total 3738 claims with total amount of ₹ 2,197.67 lakh across the seven districts in the Gulbarga division. Except Gadag, a recently created district, there are differences in average claim values, ranging between ₹ 53,402 and ₹ 61,938.

In regard to comparison of government-sponsored health insurance schemes, the people benefitted from health insurance has gone up appreciably over the years under the aegis of Rashtriya Swasthya Bima Yojna, Rajiv Aarogyasri, Vajpayee Arogyasri and Kalaignar health insurance scheme taken by the union and state governments. By an estimate, 22.3 million families were covered under RAS and Kalaignar health insurance scheme covered 13.6 million families in Tamil Nadu. Vajpayee Arogyasri Scheme covered 2.2 million families in the year 2013 and RSBY covered approximately 40.13 million BPL families across the country in January 2014. Among the government-sponsored health insurance schemes, the coverage of RSBY was the largest. All the state schemes are totally funded by the state governments but RSBY is in the ratio of 3:1 by central and state governments. Rajiv Aarogyasri Scheme and Vajpayee Arogyasri Scheme only covered chronic diseases and inpatient. RSBY covered mostly secondary care including maternity, chronic diseases and inpatient.

RSBY covered different types of healthcare packages but BPL coverage was less by the annual cap of ₹ 30,000 per family. As a result, RSBY packages covered only secondary care. The other schemes has emphasised on tertiary care with higher yearly coverage such as in RAS (₹ 150,000 per household and 50,000 sundry expenses), VAS (₹ 150,000 per household and 50,000 sundry expenses) and CMKHIS (₹ 100,000 per household for the period of four years). The coverage of RSBY was less as compared to state-sponsored schemes whereas the number of beneficiaries was greater in case of RSBY. There was huge difference in packages rates for maximum procedures under the schemes. The RSBY charged the lowest rates than the other schemes. The package rate of coronary bypass surgery was ₹ 30,000 under RSBY, ₹ 95,000 under Rajiv Aarogyasri Scheme and Vajpayee Arogyasri Scheme and ₹ 90,000 under Chief Minister Kalaignar Health Insurance Scheme which showed that RSBY has a tie up with the state governments in case of hospital empanellment, which provided the hospitalisation benefits and treated the ailments in genuine price. In other packages, it seems imperative that GSHISs should coordinate with each other to influence the price determination of services rather than serve as mere price takers. In case of packages classified by surgical and medical treatment, Gastroenterology, Ophthalmology, Ear, Nose and Throat (ENT), Obstetrics and Gynaecology (OBGYN) and general surgery, RSBY covered more packages in surgery as compared to Rajiv Aarogyasri Scheme, Chief Minister Kalaignar Health Insurance Scheme and Vajpayee Arogyasri Scheme. RSBY covered all types of in-patient care even within ₹ 30,000 as compared to other schemes. There were 11,565 hospitals under RSBY and 454 hospitals, 692 hospitals and 131 hospitals under RAS, CMKHIS and VAS schemes respectively. The maximum number of hospitals under RSBY scheme shown that the BPL population covered at large scale and there is more shining success of the scheme as compared to state schemes. The comparison of government sponsored health insurance schemes showed that RSBY provided the wide range of hospitalisation benefits to the beneficiaries across India.

5.5 Problems of Government Sponsored Health Insurance Schemes

The government-sponsored health insurance schemes is totally free to the beneficiaries. As concerned with detrimental selection will be a concern. In such situation, the more aware purchase excessive health insurance as compared to others. This can be result of paucity of information regarding health hazards faced by the beneficiary. In health-care, wide variation has been found in government-sponsored health insurance schemes (Nagpal, 2012). The reason behind the variation is that state-based health insurance schemes provide high-end, rare delivery and uncommon packages, while RSBY provides largely secondary care of regular basis with common diseases. Fraud is major hindrances in the development of health insurance sector in India where the insurers are not properly followed the rules and regulations. Two kinds of frauds are there. Sometimes the insured show lack of character and submit fictitious claims. On the other hand, the hospitals themselves commit deceit on the systems.With aim of deepening the coverage of health insurance, evolution of benefit packages is an ongoing process in response to socio-political demands, claim experience, and availability of financial resources.

Rashtriya Swasthya Bima Yojna scheme faced challenges both before and during implementation. The main challenge during the implementation of the scheme was the paper and filing work of each procedure at every stage. To clear the roles and responsibility of the stakeholders is again a challenge. At every stage the stakeholders have queries regarding the bills, claims, premiums etc. In time, this trend could make the scheme unviable. Rashtriya Swasthya Bima Yojna success which is based on the effective management, administration and implementation. According to RSBY and other state schemes enrollment data, it has been found that there is maximum listing of private providers as compared to public. Surprisingly, on the other side the private hospitals are very less in backward areas where the need is the most. It has been observed that private hospitals have an increased caseload and income whereas public hospitals have shown a decline in patients, decline in the range of functions and withdrawal of funds on the assumption that income has been generated through RSBY. The government invested in primary healthcare, but the proper facilities and availability of doctors are not up to mark.

India's system of financing healthcare is full of deficiencies. To overcome these shortcomings itself is a major challenge. Situation becomes very difficult when it has to be found that masses are poor, funds are not available in enough quantities. Healthcare is beyond BPL population reach because it is very costly. It has been found that the private expenditure is three times greater the government expenditure which leads to poverty and out-of-pocket expenses. If there would increase in public health it will balance the public and private spending which will further reduces the poverty and enhance the life style of the general public.

5.6 Policy Implications and Suggestions

On the basis of empirical analysis certain policy implications can be drawn from the study as below:

- Government of India should increase the public spending on health as a percentage of GDP which can help to mitigate the finances of public;
- In order to reach the beneficiaries, insurance companies have to approach through local self-government, non-governmental organisations (NGOs), micro finance institutions (MFIs) or other grassroot organisations to conduct information and awareness campaigns;
- The government should link RSBY with National Rural Health Mission (NRHM), National Urban Rural Health

Mission (NURHM), Panchayati Raj Institutions (PRIs) and National Rural Employment Guarantee Act (NREGA) to reach out to the grassroot level; and

- The government should introduce an Universal Health Coverage (UHC) that entitles every citizen guaranteed access to primary, secondary and tertiary healthcare services provided by public sector.

Note

1. www.rsby.gov.in

Refrences

- Adams, S., (2011), *"Health Insurance For India's Poor- Meeting the Challenge With Information Technology"*, Report Published by Deutsche Gesellschaft Fur Internationale Zusammenarbeit (GIZ), GmbH in Co-operation With India's Ministry of Labour and Employment, pp. 1-4.
- Ahuja, R., (2004), "The Poor Need Health Insurance, Too", *IRDA Journal*, 2(11), pp. 15-16.
- Ahuja, R., (2005), *"Health Insurance For The Poor In India: An Analytical Study"*, Working Paper No. 161, Indian Council for Research on International Economics Relations, June.
- Ahuja, R., and Jutting, J., (2004), *"Are The Poor Too Poor to Demand Health Insurance"*, Working Paper No. 118, Indian Council For Research on International Economics Relations, New Delhi.
- Ali, S., Mohammad, R., and Masharique, A., (2007), "*Insurance Sector in Post Liberalisation, An Impact on Legal Framework*", Insurance in India, Regal Publications, New Delhi, pp.118-124.
- Anderson, G.F., Frogner, B.K., and Reinhardt U. E., (2007), "Health Spending in OECD countries in 2004: An Update", *Health Aff (Millwood)*, 26(5), pp. 1481-89.
- Arhin-Tenkorang, D., (2000), "*Health Insurance For The Informal Sector in Africa: Design Features, Risk Protection and Resource Mobilisation"*, Working Paper No. WG 3:1, Commission on Macroeconomics and Health, Geneva.
- Arora, D., and Lipika, N., (2011), "Towards Alternative Health Financing: The Experience of RSBY in Kerala" In *India's Health Insurance Scheme for the Poor: Evidence From the Early Experience of the Rashtriya Swasthya Bima Yojna*, Centre For Policy Research, New Delhi, India.

- Bakshi, S., (2005), "Integrated Approach: Key To Growth And Development", *Vikalapa*, 30(3), pp. 108-110.
- Bajari, P., *et al.*, (2010), "Moral Hazard, Adverse Selection And Health Expenditures: A Semi-parametric Analysis", Available at http://www.econ.umn.edu/~bajari/ research/hazard.pdf (accessed November 7, 2012).
- Banga, J.S., (2007), "*Market Strategies of General Insurance Companies in India: A Study of Public Sector and Private Sector*", Ph.D. Thesis, Submitted to Punjab School of Management Studies, Punjabi University, Patiala.
- Banker, *et al.*, (1984), "Some Models for Estimating Technical and Scale Efficiency", *Management Science,* 30(6), pp.1078-1092.
- Basu, R., (2011), "*Rashtriya Swasthya Bima Yojna: Pioneering Public-Private Partnership in Health Insurance*" Paper Presented at International Conference on Relevance of Policy Reforms on Development: Challenges Before Emerging Economies, Jamia Millia Islamia (A Central University), New Delhi, India.
- Bawa, S., and Kaur, N., (2011), "Performance Measurement Using The Frontier Efficiency Methodology: A Study of Indian General Insurance Sector", *Journal of Banking, Financial Services and Insurance Research,* 1(8), pp. 49-75.
- Bawa, S., and Ruchita, (2011), "Productivity Change in the Indian Health Insurance Business: A Malmquist Total Factor Productivity Analysis", *International Journal of Research in Commerce and Management*, 2(7), pp. 115-121.
- Bearing Point Inc. (2008), "*Private Health Insurance in India: Promise and Reality",* United States Agency for International Development, New Delhi, India.
- Berman, P., and Ahuja, R., (2009), "The Impoverishing Effect of Health Care Payments in India: New Evidence and Methodology", *India Health Beat*, 2(2), pp. 1-4.
- Berg, E.S., (2009), "*Information and Health Care: A Randomized Experiment in India*", IIG Workshop, Oxford University.
- Berg, S.A., Førsund, F.R., and Jansen, E.S., (1992),"Malmquist Indices of Productivity Growth During the Deregulation of

Norwegian Banking 1980–89", *Scandinavian Journal of Economics*, 94(Supplement), pp. 211–228.

- Bhat, R., (1999), "Characteristics of Private Medical Practices in India: A Provider Prospective", *Health Policy and Planning*, 14(1), pp. 26-37.
- Bhat, R., (2005), "Insurance Industry in India: Structure, Performance and Future Challenges", *Vikalapa*, 30 (3), pp. 93-96.
- Bhat, R., and Jain, N., (2006), *"Factor Affecting the Demand for Health Insurance in a Micro Insurance Scheme"*, Research and Publications, IIM Ahmedabad, Working Paper No. 2006-07-02.
- Bhat, R., Maheshwari, S., and Saha, S., (2005), *"Third Party Administrators and Health Insurance in India: Perception of Providers and Policyholders"*, Paper Presented at Indian institute of Management, Ahmedabad.
- Bhat, R., and Babu, S., (2003), *"Health Insurance and Third Party Administrators: Issues and Challenges"*, Working Paper No. 2003-05-02, Indian Institute of Management, Ahmedabad.
- Bhatia, B.S., (1988), "*Management of Productivity in Indian Industries*" Deep and Deep Publications Pvt. Ltd., New Delhi.
- Bishnoi, V., and Saharan, R., (2007), "Health Insurance in India: Introspects and Prospects", *The ICFAI Journal of Risk and Insurance*, 4(3), pp. 58-68.
- Brown, L.D., and Amelung, V.E., (1999), "Manacled Competition: Market Reforms in German Health Care", *Health Affairs*, 18(3), pp. 76–91.
- Busse, R., (2000), "Priority-setting and Rationing in German Health Care", *Health Policy*, 50(1/2), pp. 71–90.
- Chahal, H.S., (2006), "Feasibility of Separate Health Insurance Company in India", *IRDA Journal*, 32, pp. 53-62.
- Choudhary, S., and Kiran, P., (2011), "Life Insurance Industry in India - Current Scenario", *International Journal of Management and Business Studies*, 1(3), pp. 146-150.
- Charnes, A., Cooper, W., and Rhodes, E., (1978), "Measuring Efficiency of Decision Making Unit", *European Journal of Operation Research*, 2(3), pp. 429-444.

- Cohen, *et al.*, (2009), *"Health Insurance Coverage Trends, 1959–2007: Estimates from the National Health Interview Survey"*, National Health Statistics Report, US Department of Health and Human Services, No. 17.
- Cai, J., Janvry, A., and Sadoluet, E., (2011), *"Social Networks And Insurance Take Up: Evidence From A Randomized Experiment in China"*, Research Paper No. 8, International Labour Office, Geneva.
- Cummins, J.D., Giuseppe, T., and Weiss, M.A., (1996), *"Productivity and Technical Efficiency in Italian Insurance Industry"*, The Wharton School, University of Pennsylvania, Working Paper Series -10, Presented at Georgia Productivity Seminar, Nov. 1-3, pp. 1-41.
- Cummins, J.D., and Weiss, M.A. (1998), "Analysing Firm Performance in the Insurance Industry Using Frontier Efficiency Methods", The Wharton School, University of Pennsylvania, pp. 1-45.
- Cummins, J.D., Weiss, M.A., and Zi, H. (1999), "Organisation Form and Efficiency: The Co-existence of Stock and Mutual Property Liability Insurance", *Management Science,* 45(9), pp. 1254-1269.
- Diacon, S. (2001), *"The Efficiency of U.K. General Insurance Companies"*, University of Nottingham, Centre for Risk and Insurance Studies, CRIS Discussion Paper Series 2001.111.
- Diacon, S., Starkey, K., and Brien, C. (2002), "Size and Efficiency in European Long-term Insurance Companies: An International Comparison", *The Geneva Papers on Risk and Insurance*, 27(3), pp. 444-466.
- Das, *et al.*, (2011), *"The Quality of Medical Care in India: Evidence from a Standardised Patient Study in Two States"*, World Bank Working Paper, Washington, DC.
- Dutta, S., (2012), "Evolution of Health Insurance in India- Positives and Constraints", *IRDA Journal*, 10(12), pp. 17-23.
- Desai, S., (2009), "Keeping The 'Health' in Health Insurance", *Economic and Political Weekly*, 44 (38), pp. 18-21.

- Devadasan, *et al.,* (2010), *"Performance of Community Health Insurance in India: Findings From Empirical Studies"*, At First National Conference on Bringing Evidence Into Public Health Policy, Bangalore, India.
- Devadasan, N., (2006), "Health Financing: Protecting the Poor", *Indian Journal of Community Medicine*, 31(1), pp. 107-110.
- Devadasan, N., and Nandraj S., (2006), *"Planning & Implementing Health Insurance Programmes in India"*, Institute of Public Health, Bangalore, India.
- Devadasan, *et al.,* (2004), "Community Insurance in India: An Overview", *Economic and Political Weekly*, 39(28), pp. 3179-83.
- Diacon, S., (2001), *"The Efficiency of UK General Insurance Companies"*, Centre for Risk and Insurance Studies, Discussion paper series-2001.3, The University of Nottingham, Available at (http://www.nottingham.ac .uk/ business / cris/papers/2001-03.pdf assessed on 2.5.2010).
- Dhingra, R., (2001), "NGOs and Health Insurance Schemes in India", *Health and Population - Perspectives and Issues,* 24(4), pp. 206-217.
- Dilip, T.R., (2012), "On Publically Financed Health Insurance Schemes. Is the Analysis Premature?", *Economic and Political Weekly*, 47(18), pp. 79-80.
- Donni, O., and Fecher, F., (1997), "Efficiency and Productivity of the Insurance Industry in the OECD Countries", *The Geneva Papers on Risk and Insurance*, 22(84), July, pp. 525-535.
- Drechsler, D., and Jutting, J., (2007), "The Role of Private Health Insurance in Developing Countries", *Journal of Health Politics, Policy and Law*, 32(3), pp. 497-534.
- Dror, et al., (2008), "Cost of Illness:Evidence from a Study in Five Resource-Poor Locations in India", The *Indian Journal of Medical Research,* 127(4), pp. 347-61.
- Dutta, S., (2012), "Evolution of Health Insurance in India- Positives and Constraints", *IRDA Journal*, 10(12), pp. 17-23.
- Einav, L., Amy, F., Stephen, R., Paul, S., and Mark, R. C., (2011), *"Selection on Moral Hazard in Health Insurance",* National Bureau of Economic Research, Working Paper, 16969.

- Economy watch (2011), *"India's Universal Health Insurance Scheme"*, Available At <http://www.economywatch.com/indianeconomy/universal-health-insurance scheme.html>, Accessed on November 15.
- Ellis, R.P., Alam, M., and Gupta, I., (2000), "Health Insurance in India: Prognosis and Prospectus", *Economic and Political Weekly*, 35(4), pp. 207-217.
- European Productivity Agency (1955), "*Productivity Measurement*", Organisation for European Economic Co-operation, Paris, Vol. 1.
- Fan, V., and Mahal, A., (2011), "Learning and Getting Better: Rigorous Evaluation of Health Policy in India", *The National Medical Journal of India*, 24(6), pp. 325-327.
- Farrell, M. J., (1957), "The Measurement of Productive Efficiency", *Journal of Royal Statistical Society, Series A (General),* 120(3), pp. 253-290.
- Flores, G., Krishnakumar, J., O'Donne,l O., and Eddy, V.D., (2008), "Coping with Health Care Costs: Implications for the Measurement of Catastrophic Expenditure and Poverty", *Health Economics*, 17(12), pp. 1393-412.
- Forgia, G., and Nagpal, S., (2012), "*Government Sponsored Health Insurance in India Are You Covered?*", Washington, D.C., World Bank.
- Garg, M.C., and Deepti (2008), "Efficiency of General Insurance Industry in India in the Post-Liberalisation Era: A Data Envelopment Approach", *The ICFAI Journal of Risk and Insurance,* 5(1), pp. 32-49.
- Gudwani, *et al.,* (2012), *"India Healthcare: Inspiring Possibilities Challenging Survey"*, Report of Confederation of Indian Industry Prepared by Mckinsey and Company.
- Gupta, A., (2004), "Wealth Through Health Insurance", *IRDA Journa*l, 2(11), pp. 24-25.
- Gupta, A., (2013), "Health Insurance- The Next Paradigm", *IRDA Journal*, 11(6), pp. 15-20.

- Gumber, A., and Kulkarani, V., (2000), "Health Insurance for Informal Sector Case Study of Gujarat", *Economic and Political Weekly*, 35(40), pp. 3607-3613.
- GOI (2004), *"National Common Minimum Programme of the Government of India"*, New Delhi, India.
- Government of India (2010), *"National Health Policy 2002"*, Availablee At mohfw.nic.in/NRHM/Documents/National Health Policy 2002 pdf., Accessed On October 12, 2010.
- GOI, (2011), "*Annual Report 2010-11*", Ministry of Finance, Government of India.
- GOI (2012), "*Annual Report 2011-12*", Ministry of Finance, Government of India.
- Harris, R., Kip, R., and Snook, T., (2004), "The Foundation is Numbers – Three Requirements for Health Insurance in India", *IRDA Journal*, 2(11), pp. 30-32.
- Helms, R., (2008), *"Tax Policy and the History of Health Insurance Industry"*, Presented at Conference Taxes and Health Insurance: Analysis and Policy at Brookings Institution, Washington, D.C.
- Hjalmarsson, L., and Veiderpass, A., (1992) "Efficiency and Ownership in Swedish Electricity Retail Distribution", *Journal of Productivity Analysis,* 3(1), pp. 7–23.
- Hsiao, W., (1995), "The Chinese Health Care System: Lessons For Other Nations", *Social Science & Medicine*, Vol. 41(8), pp.1047-1055.
- IBEF (2010), *"Annual Report"*, India Brand Equity Foundation, New Delhi.
- ILO (1996), "*World Development Report 1996/1997*", International Labour Organisation, Geneva.
- IIMA (1999), "*Health Insurance in India*", Report of the One Day Workshop at Indian Institute of Management, Ahmedabad on October 30.
- IIMA (2000), "*Health Insurance*", Report on Conference on March 18-19, 2000 and Three Technical Workshops on March 15-17 at Indian Institute of Management, Ahmedabad.

- IRDA (2002), "*Protection of Policyholders' Interest 2002*", Insurance Regulatory and Development Authority, New Delhi, India.
- IRDA (2004), "*Annual Report 2003-04*", Insurance Regulatory and Development Authority, New Delhi, India.
- IRDA (2010), "*Annual Report 2009-10*", Insurance Regulatory and Development Authority, New Delhi, India.
- IRDA (2012), "*Annual Report 2011-12*", Insurance Regulatory and Development Authority, New Delhi, India.
- IRDA (2013), "*Guidelines on Standardisation*", Insurance Regulatory and Development Authority, New Delhi, India.
- IRDA (2013), "*Handbook on Insurance Repository*", Insurance Regulatory and Development Authority, New Delhi, India.
- IRDA (2013), *"Annual Report 2012-13"*, Insurance Regulatory and Development Authority, New Delhi, India.
- IRDA (2007), "*History of insurance in India*", Available At http://www.irda.gov.in/ADMINCMS/cms/NormalData_Layout.aspx?page=PageNo4&mid=2
- IRDA Regulations (2012), "*Exposure Draft- Health Insurance Regulations*", Insurance Regulatory and Development Authority, New Delhi, India.
- IIB (2008), "Annual Report 2007-08", Insurance Information Bureau of India, Bangalore, India.
- IIB (2009), "Annual Report 2008-09", Insurance Information Bureau of India, Bangalore, India.
- IIB (2010), "Annual Report 2009-10", Insurance Information Bureau of India, Bangalore, India.
- IIB (2011), "Annual Report 2010-11", Insurance Information Bureau of India, Bangalore, India.
- IIB (2012), "Annual Report 2011-12", Insurance Information Bureau of India, Bangalore, India.
- Jeng, V., and Lai, G.C. (2005), "Ownership Structure, Agency Costs, Specialisation and Efficiency: Analysis of Keiretsu and Independent Insurance Industry", *The Journal of Risk and Insurance,* 72(1), pp. 105-138.

- James, C. P., (2004), "Covering the Poorest", *IRDA Journal*, Vol. 2(11), pp. 17-21.
- Jaswal, M., (2010), "Insuring Health of Millions-Smart Use of Technology", *IRDA Journal*, 8(12), pp. 25-28.
- Kaur, N., and Kapoor, R., (2007), "Profitability Analysis of Public Sector Banks in India", *Indian Management Studies Journal,* 11, pp. 167-181.
- Kannan, N., and Thangavel, N., (2008), "Overview of Indian Insurance Sector", *Academic Open Internet Journal*, 22, ISSN 1311-4360.
- Kumar, S., and Gulati, R., (2008), "An Examination Of Technical, Pure Technical and Scale Efficiencies in Indian Public Sector Banks Using Data Envelopment Analysis", *Eurasian Journal Of Business and Economics*, 1(2), pp. 33-69.
- Kawachi, I., Wilkimon, R., and Kennedy, (1999), "*The Society and Population Health Reader*", Income Inequality and Health, New Press, New York.
- Klien, R., (1995), "*The New Politics of the National Health Service*", New York, Longman.
- Lenaghan, J., (1997), "*Hard Choices in Health Care – Rights and Rationing in Europe*", London: BMJ Publishing Group, pp. 21-47.
- Leontief, W.W., (1963), "*Studies in the Structure of American Economy*", Oxford University Press, New York.
- Matthies, S., and Cahill, R. K., (2004), "Lessons From Across The World- How Indians Can Break Barriers to Develop Health Insurance", *IRDA Journal,* 2(11), pp. 7-12.
- Mathur, P.N., (1963), "An Efficient Path of Technological Transformation of an Economy", In Barna, T. (ed.), *Structural Dependence and Economic Development*, Macmillan.
- Mali, P., (1978), "*Improving Total Factor Productivity, MBO Strategies for Business, Government And Not For Profit Organisation*", John Wiley and Sons, Inc.
- Malvankar, D., and Bhat, R., (2000), "*Health Insurance in India: Opportunities, Challenges and Concerns*", Paper Presented at Indian Institute of Management, Ahmedabad.

- Mahal, A., (2000), "Assessing Private Health Insurance in India: Potential impacts and Regulatory Issues", *Economic and Political Weekly*, 37(6), pp. 559-71.
- Miller, M.D., and Schmidt, J.W., (1984), *"Industrial Engineering and Operation Research"*, John Wiley and Sons, Inc. Canada, pp. 436.
- Majumdar, P., (2004), "Back to the Actuary- Thoughts on How Health Insurance Should Grow", *IRDA Journal*, 2(11), pp. 28-29.
- Mahal, A., (2002), "Assessing Private Health Insurance in India: Potential Impacts and Regulatory Issues", *Economic and Political Weekly*, 37(6), pp. 559-71.
- Maheshwari, S., (2005), "Managing Insurance: Managing the Agents", *Vikalapa*, 30(3), pp. 115-119.
- Mathiyazhagan, K., (1998), "Willingness to Pay Through Community Participation in India", *The International Journal of Health Planning and Management*, 13(1), pp. 47-67.
- Mansor, S.A., and Radam, A., (2000), "Productivity and Efficiency Performance of the Malaysian Life Insurance Industry", *Journal Economy Malaysia,* 34(2000), pp. 93-105.
- Ministry of Labour and Employment (2009), "*Project Information Document (PID) Concept Stage*", Government of India, Report No. AB3988.
- Mony, S., (2005), "New Initiatives in the Insurance Sector: Opportunities and Challenges", *Vikalapa*, 30(3), pp. 102-105.
- MOHFW (2011), "*Framework For Developing Health Insurance Programmes*", Ministry of Health and Family Welfare, Government of India, New Delhi.
- MOHFW (2012), *"Annual Report"*, Ministry of Health and Family Welfare, Government of India, New India.
- Ministry of Health and Family Welfare (2012), *"Performance Audit of the Implementation of the National Rural Health Mission"*, Comptroller and Auditor General of India, New Delhi, India.
- MOHFW (2002), *"National Health Policy"*, Ministry of Health and Family Welfare, New Delhi, India.

- NSSO (2004), *"Morbidity Health Care and Condition of Aged"*, Report No. 507, Jan-June.
- Narayanan, H., (2006), "*Indian Insurance and Globalisation*", Indian Insurance: A Profile, Jaico Publishing House, Mumbai, pp. 94-101.
- Nagendranath, A., and Chari, P., (2002), *"Health Insurance in India: The Emerging Paradigms"*, Paper Presented at 'Insurance '02": A seminar on the Emerging Issues on the Indian Insurance Sector At IIFT- School of International Business Management, New Delhi.
- Nagpal S., Devdasan, N., and Jain, N., (2007), "Health Security For all- Government Initiatives in Health Insurance", *IRDA Journal*, 6(2), pp. 25-30.
- Nakamura (2001), *"Establishment of the Partnership Between Southeast Asian Countries in the Field of Public Health and Medical Services"*, NIRA E ASIA Research team ed.
- NCEUS (2007), "*Report on Conditions of Work and Promotion of Livelihoods in the Unorganised Sector"*, National Commission for Enterprises in the Unorganised Sector, Government of India, New Delhi.
- Newhouse, J., (1996), "Reimbursing Health Plans and Health Providers: Efficiency in Production Versus Selection", *Journal Of Economic Literature*, 34(3), pp.1236-63.
- Outreville, J. F., (1991), "*Use of Computer Technology in the Insurance Sector of Developing Countries*", Discussion Paper 38, United Nations Conference on Trade and Development, Geneva.
- Parasuraman, A., Zeithaml, V.A., and Berry, L.L. (1994), "Reassessment of Expectations as a Comparison Standard in Measuring Service Quality: Implications For Further Research", *Journal of Marketing,* 58, pp.111-124.
- Peters, *et al.,* (2002), *"Better Health Systems for India's Poor: Findings, Analysis and Options"*, Health, Nutrition and Population Series, Washington D.C., World Bank.
- Planning Commission of India (2007), "*Poverty Estimates for 2004–05*", Press Information Bureau, Government of India, New Delhi.

- Planning Commission of India (2011), "*Faster, Sustainable and More Inclusive Growth*", 12th Five Year Plan Approach Paper 2012–17, Planning Commission of India, Government of India, New Delhi.
- Preker, A., Langeubrunner, J., and Jakab, M., (2002), "*Rich-Poor Differences in Health Care Financing*", In: Dror D, Preker A, Editors, Washington, D.C., World Bank.
- Price, C.W. and Weyman-Jones, T., (1996), "Malmquist Indices of Productivity Change in the UK Gas Industry Before and After Privatisation", *Applied Economics,* 28(1), pp. 29-39.
- Rajan, A.K., and Dhunna, M., (2002), "Liberalisation of Insurance Sector: Social Implications", *Indian Management Studies Journal,* 6(1), April, pp.109-118.
- Rao, R.S.B., (2004), "Medical Policies for the Masses- The Surging Need For Pan-population Health Insurance", *IRDA Journal,* 2(11), pp. 13-14.
- Rao, G., and Choudhary, M., (2012), *"Health Care Financing Reforms in India"*, Working Paper No. 2012-100, National Institute of Public Finance and Policy, pp. 1-13.
- Rao, S. *et al.,* (2005), *"Financing and Delivery of Health Care Services in India"*, National Commission on Macroeconomics and Health, Ministry of Health and Family Welfare, Government of India, New Delhi.
- Ranson, K., and Jowett, M., (2003), "*Developing Health Insurance in India: Background Paper to the Government of India*", Workshop on Health Insurance.
- Ravisankar, T.S., (1996), "Managerial Challenge: Review of Reforms", *IBA Bulletin* 18(1), pp. 80-84.
- Reddy, *et al.,* (2011), "Towards achievement of Universal Health Care in India By 2020: A Call To Action" *Lancet,* 377(9767), pp. 760-68.
- Saltman, R.B., Figueras, J.U., and Sakellarides, C., (1998), "*Critical Challenges for Health Care Reform in Europe*", Open University Press, Buckingham.
- Savedoff, W. D., (2008), *"Governing Mandatory Health Insurance: Concepts, Framework, and Cases"*, In Learning from

Experience: Governing Mandatory Health Insurance, Washington, D.C., World Bank.

- Seiford, L. M., and Zhu, J., (1999), "An Investigation of Returns-to-scale in Data Envelopment Analysis", *Omega*, 27(1), pp. 1-11.
- Segal, M., (2004), "Prescribed: Growth Tonics - Private Health insurance in Dire Need of Fillip", *IRDA Journal*, 2(11), pp. 26-27.
- Selvaraj, S., and Karan, A.K., (2012), "Why Publicly- Financed Health Insurance Schemes are Ineffective in Providing Financial Risk Protection", *Economic and Political Weekly*, 47(11): 61-68.
- Selvaraj, S., and Nabar, V., (2010), "*Access to Medicines in India: Issues, Challenges and Response*", India Health Report, Business Standard Limited, New Delhi, pp. 83-96.
- Selvavinayagam, T.S., and Kumar, V., (2012), "Overview of Publicly funded Health Insurance : Tamil Nadu Model", *Indian Journal of Community Medicine,* 37(3), pp. 194-196.
- Sharma, M.K., and Agarwal, P., (2005), "Globalisation of Indian Insurance Sector – The Emerging Scenario", *Indian Management Studies Journal*, 9(2) pp. 47-58.
- Shijith, V.P., and Sekher, T.V., (2011), "*Who Gets Health Insurance Coverage in India? : New Findings From Nation-wide Surveys*", 27, IUSSP International Population Conference Busan, Korea.
- Shukla, T., (2007), "Health Insurance Industry in India: Prospects and Challenges", *Journal of Marketing Trends*, 1(1), pp. 26-38.
- Shinde, G., Patil D.Y., and Bhalerao, K., (2011), "Journey of Insurance Sector in India: Since Its Inception", *Indian Streams Research Journal*, 1(4), pp.1-8.
- Sihare, H., and Sihare, M., (2010), "Pharmaceutical Financing For Below Poverty Line Through Micro Health Insurance: Health For All", *Pharmacophore*, 1(2), pp. 45-64.
- Sinha, R.P., (2006), "Operating Efficiency of Life Insurance Companies: A Data Envelopment Approach", *The ICFAI Journal of Risk and Insurance,* 3(4), pp. 29-37.
- Sinha, R., (2007), "Productivity and Efficiency of Indian General Insurance Industry," *Journal of Risk and Insurance*, 4(2), pp. 33-43.

- Sinha, T., (2004), "*The Indian Insurance Industry: Challenges and Prospects*", Swiss Re Sigma Report of Institute of Insurance and Risk Management.
- Sinha, T., (2005), "*An Analysis of the Evolution of Insurance in India", Centre For Risk And Insurance Studies,* Discussion Paper Series-III, pp. 1-68.
- Singh, D., (2011), *"A Study on the Development of Health Insurance – Its History, Current Scenario and Future Prospects in India"*, D. Subramanian Award With Report Presented.
- Singh, I., and Kumar, P., (2005), "Efficiency Analysis: The Case of Indian Banking Industry", *The Indian Economic Journal*, 52(3-4), pp. 133-138.
- Srinivasan, R., (2001), "Health Insurance in India", *Health and Population Perspectives and Issues*, 24 (2), pp. 65-72.
- Sodani, P.R., (2001), *"Potential of Health Insurance for Informal Sector: A Pilot Study"*, Indian Institute of Health Management Research, Jaipur- Rajasthan, India.
- Soderlund, N., and Hans l, B., (2000), "Health Insurance in South Africa: An Empirical Analysis of Trends in Risk Pooling and Efficiency Following Deregulation", *Health Policy and Planning*, 15(4), pp. 378-385.
- Swarup, A., (2008), *"Rashtriya Swasthya Bima Yojna- Providing Health Insurance Cover to the Poor"*, Presented at Asia-Pacific Regional High-Level Meeting on Socially-Inclusive Strategies to Extend Social Security Coverage, New Delhi, India.
- Swarup, A., and Jain, N., (2011), *"Rashtriya Swasthya Bima Yojna: A Case Study From India"*, Paper Selected By ILO and UNDP.
- Thakur and Kumar (2013), "Health Insurance Penetration in India: Implications For Marketers", *International Journal of Advances in Engineering Sciences*, 3(3), pp. 121-124.
- USAID (2010), "*Rashtriya Swasthya Bima Yojna 2010 Guide book*", A Joint Initiative of USAID and Mission Convergence, GNCTD.
- Vashisht, S., and Pandit, N., (2012), "Experiences of RSBY Beneficiaries in a District of Western India – A Qualitative Study",

International Journal of Economics and Management Review, 2(7), pp. 1-8.

- Vellakkal, S., (2009), "*Adverse Selection and Private Health Insurance Coverage in India: A Rational Behaviour Model of Insurance Agents Under Asymmetric Information*", Working Paper No. 233, Indian Council for Research on International Economic Relations, New Delhi, India.
- Verma *et al.*, (2013), "Health Insurance: Need of the Hour in India", *International Journal of Basic and Applied Medical Sciences*", 3(2), pp. 161-165.
- Vyasalu, V., (2008), "The Case Against Health Insurance', *Economic and Political Weekly*, 43(39), pp. 3495-97.
- Wagstaff, A., Lindelow, M., Junc, G., Ling, X., and Juncheng, Q., (2009), "Extending Health Insurance to the Rural Population: An Impact Evaluation of China's New Cooperative Medical Scheme", *Journal of Health Economics*, 28, pp. 1-19.
- World Bank (1993), "*World Development Report: Investing in Health*", Oxford University Press, Washington, D.C., World Bank.
- World Bank (2008), "*Governing Mandatory Health Insurance: Learning From Experience*", Washington, D.C., World Bank.
- WHO (1997), "*Highlights on Health in the Netherlands*", WHO Regional Office For Europe.
- WHO (2010), "*World Health Statistics, 2010*", Geneva, World Health Organisation.
- WHO (2009), "*World Health Statistics 2009*", cited 2010, http://www.who.int/whosis/whostat/2009/en/index.
- World Health Organisation (1987), "*Evaluation of the Strategy For Health For All By The Year 2000*", Geneva.
- World Health Organisation, (2000), "*The Economic Impacts of Tuberculosis*", The Stop TB Initiative 2000 Series, Geneva.
- Worthington, A., (1999), "Malmquist Indices of Productivity Change in Australian Financial Services", *Journal of International Financial Markets, Institutions and Money*, 9(3), pp. 303-320.
- Yip, W., Hong, W., and Yuanli, L., (1998), "Determinants of Patient Choice of Medical Provider: A Case Study in Rural China", *Health Policy and Planning*, 13(3), pp. 311-322.

- Yellaiah, J., (2013), "Health Insurance in India: Rajiv Aarogyasri Health Insurance Scheme in Andhra Pradesh", *IOSR Journal of Humanities and Social Science,* 8(1), pp.7-14.
- www.aarogyasri.org
- www.districts.nic.in
- www.healthcare.com
- www.ifmr.ac.in
- www.irdaindia.org
- www.iphindia.org
- www.ilo.org
- www.nottingham.ac.uk
- www.rsby.in
- www.sas.gov.in
- www.tnhsp.org
- www.whoindia.org

Index